Medications for Anxiety & Depression

A no-nonsense, comprehensive guide to the most common (and not so common) antidepressants and anti-anxiety drugs available

2015 Updated Edition

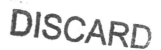

Benjamin Kramer

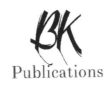

Publications

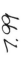

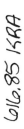

Important Disclaimer

Contents

Introduction

It is unfortunate that there remains a pervasive stigma associated with taking drugs to treat mood disorders. Sometimes this negative view of drugs comes from those who know someone taking medication. They may think that you are "crazy" or "unstable" if you take medication, causing them to tiptoe around the topic, thereby creating an uncomfortable elephant in the room. However, more problematic is the bias against drugs which exists in the sufferer themselves.

It pains me to imagine the unnecessary suffering which occurs across the entire planet because people with a mood disorder refuse to consider medication in cases where there would be immense benefit. Some people worry that it will change their personality; that they will be "high on drugs", that they will become a zombie and many other mostly unfounded reasons. In my experience, the most common manifestation of this problem is in patients who are strictly "all natural", favouring alternative therapies, eschewing "Big Pharma". I have a lot of experience with this demographic as I often promote the use of non-drug treatments for certain conditions, such as my long-time love of supplements such as curcumin or milk thistle. People are sometimes shocked to discover that I recommend the use of pharmaceutical medication in certain cases, expecting me to be a fervent anti-drug zealot.

In fact, I am neither anti-drug nor anti-natural therapies. I am stridently non-fundamentalist, believing in the right treatment for the right condition. So while I believe that many people refuse medication which would drastically improve their anxiety, I also believe that just as many (if not more – especially in western countries) are put on medication unnecessarily.

This is an incredibly complex topic. Covering its every nuance would be beyond the scope of this guide as there are just so many factors at play. For example, many people don't realise that the prevalence of drug-based therapies is partly economic. It would be extremely expensive for governments or insurance companies to pay for long term non-drug therapies such as CBT. It is much cheaper just to hand someone a prescription for an SSRI or a benzodiazepine and hope they get better.

Prescription pharmaceuticals play a central role in treating depression and anxiety for a good reason – they are relatively cheap and effective. That said, they are undoubtedly over-prescribed in many cases, often being the first line of treatment for mild cases which would be better suited to non-pharmacological treatments such as cognitive behavioural therapy (CBT) or exercise therapy. However, at the end of the day, for the majority of people, they *do* work.

Please don't allow yourself be unduly influenced by scare-mongering on the internet, whether by 'alternative' practitioners telling you that antidepressants cause 'brain damage' (if they did, they wouldn't still be available after all this time) or by reading comments on internet forums. Remember, internet forums are a classic example of *selection bias*. People most likely to hang around depression and anxiety forums are those who are not being helped by their medication. If you get sick, take your medication and get better, you will just get on with your life and will be highly unlikely to go on these forums[1]. The other way to verify for yourself is to talk to any close friends or relatives who have used antidepressants and to get their first-hand views.

The purpose of this guide is to equip you with the key information to enable you to make the right choices when it comes to the selection of the appropriate medication for your particular situation. In consultation with your doctor, you should take an active role in deciding on the best treatment. Unfortunately, this topic is littered with misunderstandings and half-truths, so hopefully I can help you go some way towards helping you make the right choices.

In order to identify the medications with the highest probability of working for you, you will need to understand the basics of neurochemistry and neuroscience in general. The other night when I returned home from work, there was nobody home so all the lights were out. I fumbled through the various keys on my keychain, trying to work out which one was my door key based on how they felt. I then tried poking around in the general vicinity of the lock, trying to find the keyhole. After having no success, I eventually turned on the flashlight app on my phone, finding the right key and then the keyhole in moments. Much of the time, this is how patients (and even some doctors) approach the selection of psychotropic medication.

So I recommend you first shine a light on your brain and mind to locate the keyhole. Then you can identify the right key to fit this keyhole. Unfortunately, much of the time, when people first visit their doctor, after a hurried, cursory discussion, they leave the doctor's office with a prescription for the same SSRI or benzodiazepine which that particular doctor gives all their patients with mood disorders. As you will have received a "key" without the doctor understanding what the "keyhole" looks like, your recovery may hinge on pure chance rather than targeted therapy. I have no doubt that this is one of the major drivers behind the reason why so many patients fail to recover after starting their first drug.

However, in order to do this, you will need to know what to look for, which is why I want to first cover some of the fundamental aspects of the story such as the various neurotransmitters which influence mood and anxiety. Depression involving low serotonin can look dramatically different to depression involving low dopamine. Depending on whether serotonin or dopamine is your issue (let alone the other neurotransmitters) the right medication may be completely different.

---

[1] The exception here is the wonderful sub-group of people who decide to remain on forums until after they are "well" to provide guidance and moral support to others. These people are saints in my view.

At this juncture, if there is one piece of vital information I can give you it is to ensure you are referred to a clinical psychiatrist. General practitioners and family doctors do a wonderful job, however they are required to act as "jack of all trades", with a little bit of knowledge on a wide range of common health complaints. Properly trained psychiatrists however, not only know a lot more about mood disorders (and can therefore identify common problems and the best pharmaceutical solution) they have extensive clinical experience with a large number of patients. They know what works and what doesn't. This means they are not prescribing based on just marketing materials received from drug companies. If you believed the pre-release and marketing information on drugs like reboxetine or agomelatine, you would think that they are the panacea for all mood disorders. Fortunately your psychiatrist will know whether this is actually true or not, based on clinical experience. Another key point here is that your psychiatrist will therefore be more comfortable trying off-label or treatment-resistant options. Many primary care providers are uncomfortable prescribing anything except SSRIs. Too many times I have seen a patient simply rotated across the various SSRIs, despite the fact that their condition warranted a more tailored approach.

My aim is to keep things 'to the point' and stick to the key facts only. No-one needs another 500 page book on neuroscience – there are enough of those already. This guide will look at the major pharmaceuticals available for the treatment of anxiety, depression and related conditions such as fibromyalgia. It will also look at the slight variations in these conditions which require differing treatments, along with some possible combinations of different classes of medication.

As I always say, don't diagnose yourself using a book or a web-site. There are simply too many individual variables which need to be considered, requiring face to face expert attention. However my general rule of thumb is that mild to moderate cases of anxiety or depression can usually be treated without the use of drugs, whereas more severe cases almost always benefit from the addition of one or more drugs. That said, one thing I always caution against is simply taking a pill, sitting back and expecting it to do all the work. If someone starts taking a drug to treat their anxiety, they should also work to address whatever it was that made them anxious in the first place. Not only will this turbo-charge a person's recovery, it can often lead to a complete remission, enabling the person to eventually come off their medication.

In the first edition of this book, I created a section at the end where I listed a number of strategies, core principles and repeating themes. For this new edition, I have instead decided to weave these ideas more naturalistically throughout the book as the situation warrants, so that each concept arises in close proximity to a useful, real-world application.

I know this guide has helped many people already and I hope it also provides you with some clarity around which direction to head on the path to recovery, repair and restoration *(Don't worry, that will be the only time in the book I make an amateurish attempt at alliteration!)*.

When I first wrote guide several years ago, there was one relatively unknown off-label antidepressant which I had begun researching. However at that time I wasn't yet comfortable mentioning it until I had built up some more real world (meaning, first hand, from patients) experience. In this time there has also been an explosion of research into this drug via studies and clinical trials. This is not a new drug. It has simply been used to treat other conditions, with experts only recently discovering that it can also act as a potent antidepressant and anti-anxiety agent.

It would be an understatement to say that I have been astounded at the life-changing effects this drug has had for some people. That's not to say that it works as a universal panacea. It doesn't work for everyone, but when it does work, boy oh boy does it work powerfully. The interesting part is that it works via a mechanism entirely unrelated to other antidepressants. In fact, apart from some minor and incidental antagonism of one of the serotonin receptor sub-types, it essentially leaves serotonin untouched. Later in the book I will explain why I think this is incredibly interesting.

I won't mention it by name until the end of the guide as I don't want it clouding your assessment of the more commonly available drugs such as SSRIs, so please don't cheat by skipping ahead. There is a method to my madness. SSRIs should still remain the first choice for many people – at least until there are more trials and a greater sample size to draw from. Imagine you have lost your car keys and there are around ten or so places you might have left them. Naturally you would start looking in the most likely places and then, via a process of elimination, move sequentially down the list. Your keys *might* be in one of the less likely spots, however more often than not, they will most likely be where you thought they would. For most people, SSRIs are the first place they should probably look. However, if you have eliminated the most likely places to look, this drug I am talking about may give you one extra place to look. And the fascinating part is that it is in a place you least expect.

A Basic Overview

Before we move on to specific medications, I think it would be useful to look at the different ways you can reduce depression and anxiety pharmacologically. For so many people, their medication is like a "black box". Their psychiatrist tells them what they need and then they obediently take the drug, no questions asked. For many people, this is just how they like it. After all, they are often in this predicament due to a stressful life with a multitude of commitments – the last thing they want is to take an active role in choosing or even understanding what exactly is going on "under the hood" when they take their medication. If this describes you, that's completely fine, however if possible, I recommend people at least familiarize themselves with some of the general categories and principles.

This is a perfect example of that common expression – *knowledge is power*. Chances are you will require a few tweaks and changes as your doctor calibrates your treatment to arrive at the best possible option. The more you understand about each class of drug, their risks and side-effects, how long they take to start working and a range of other factors, the more you will be able to provide your doctor with useful feedback and manage your own expectations.

So before we cover each category of medication and the individual drugs within each category, I wanted to distil some of the core principles down to the basics for those unfamiliar with the pharmacology of anxiety disorders.

GABA (gamma amino butyric acid)

GABA is the primary "calming" or *inhibitory* neurotransmitter in your brain, putting the brake on mental activity, including anxiety. As GABA is like your brain's "master switch", it is the quickest and most powerful pathway to reducing anxiety. GABA works by activating GABA receptors, which then inhibits the transmission of certain signals around the brain, causing anxiety to subside. The main way that certain medications use the GABA pathway to reduce anxiety is by artificially activating (*agonising*) GABA receptors. This contrasts with drugs like Prozac, which work by boosting the availability of the neurotransmitter (serotonin in the case of Prozac) itself.

If you have visited a supplement retailer looking for "natural" supplements for anxiety, you may have seen GABA advertised as a product. I have serious issues with the ethics of this, as these supplement manufacturers would know that GABA has a poor ability to cross the blood brain barrier (BBB), which is like a filter that prevents certain substances or large molecules from entering (and perhaps damaging) your brain. So if you took GABA as a pill, it would be digested and then enter the blood stream, however would not reach the brain. There is a good reason why there are no major anti-anxiety medications which work by simply taking GABA as a pill. This is the same reason why there is no antidepressant which is just serotonin in a pill (serotonin has the same problem with the BBB, so the closest you can get is the amino acid l-tryptophan or the supplement 5-htp, both of which are the building blocks of serotonin).

The easiest way to look at it is – more GABAergic activity, less anxiety. GABA is one of the easier neurotransmitters to understand in this sense. With other neurotransmitters, it is not as simple as increasing or decreasing activity. For example, dopamine is the neurotransmitter of pleasure, however if dopamine activity is pushed too high, schizophrenic-style symptoms such as hallucinations can result.

A drug can also influence the activity of GABA via indirect means. As GABA is such a major player, there are two way connections with a multitude of other neurotransmitters and receptors. Which leads me to glutamate, the "yin" to GABA's "yang". [2]

Of the various forms of mood disorders, GABA tends to be a central player in anxiety disorders, playing only a minor role in depression. In fact, GABA's

---

[2] Or should it be the other way around? Sorry, Taoism is not my strong suit!

relationship with mood can be tricky. For example, if you had chronic anxiety caused by a lack of GABAergic activity (either directly or due to out of control glutamate activity), it is likely that this will eventually lead to depression for many people. So in this sense, a functioning GABA system is important. However on the flip-side, taking drugs such as benzodiazepines at high doses or long term can be a factor in the development of depression. This is yet another example of the nuance involved, demonstrating why a careful, considered approach is always warranted.

After spending several decades under the spell of serotonin, recently researchers have been focusing at lot of attention on glutamate, and in particular one type of glutamatergic receptor – the NMDA receptor. Because glutamate is central to a whole host of brain functions, by modulating it, downstream effects occur which can be potently anxiolytic or anti-depressive. I firmly believe that in ten years, drugs which act on glutamate will be central to the treatment of mood disorders. I cover this in extensive detail a bit later.

Glutamate (GLUT)

If GABA is the "brakes", glutamate is the brain's main "accelerator". However the relationship between GABA and glutamate is significantly more complex than this simplified analogy. Sometimes when people first read about glutamate being *excitatory*, they imagine that it gives you energy, like caffeine or amphetamines. Whilst this may be the case, depending on how a drug influences glutamate, it would be more accurate to describe this yin/yang pair like this – Imagine your brain needs to send a message from one side to the other. If GABA dominates at this particular point in time or a particular part of the brain, it inhibits the message from being transmitted. If glutamate dominates, the message will most likely reach its destination.

A good practical example of this is where someone suffers from epilepsy or other types of seizures. This involves uncontrolled glutamate-driven brain activity – like an electrical storm in your head. Unsurprisingly, most anti-seizure drugs work by boosting the activity of GABA or suppressing the activity of glutamate. You can make your car go slower by either taking your foot off the accelerator or pressing down on the brakes.

Generally speaking, most mood disorders involve the foot being pushed too hard on the accelerator, or alternatively, brakes which are not working properly. When the GABA/glutamate relationship is working well, as part of this "yin/yang" aspect, each keeps the other in check. This is achieved via the way they are synthesised, as GABA can be used to make glutamate and the other way around. Imagine you need to split a million dollars in $50 notes with your business partner. As you are making two piles, when one pile gets clearly taller than the other, you can take from one and give to the smaller pile, so each pile is contributing to this evening out process.

Serotonin

Serotonin is an incredibly complex neurotransmitter with a diverse range of effects throughout the brain and body. You may have read about serotonin as being the "happy" neurotransmitter, with the implication that all you need to do is boost serotonin and all your troubles will melt away. It is correct to say that, in general, more serotonergic activity equals less anxiety and depression (After all, as the author of a book called *Increase Serotonin Naturally*, to state otherwise would be inconsistent of me, to say the least!). However in reality, serotonin's effects are much more complex than a simple "less serotonin = depression/anxiety" equation.

This can be tricky when treating mood disorders. For example, drugs which boost serotonergic activity can have the effect of suppressing dopamine activity. This is great for disorders like generalised anxiety disorder (GAD) or panic disorder, but less so for social anxiety, which can require a boost in dopamine to give you confidence in social settings. And considering the relationship between dopamine and your ability to feel pleasure, suppressed dopaminergic activity can also be a factor in depression.

This is further complicated by the large number of different sub-types of serotonin receptors. Activating some of them can cause anxiety or depression to decrease, whereas others have the opposite effect. I will cover this in greater detail when I look at drugs which modulate serotonin.

Serotonin can be tricky in terms of finding your "sweet spot". For example, if you take too high a dose of a serotonin-boosting drug, you may find your anxiety has disappeared but so too has your motivation, ability to feel pleasure and sex drive, because of serotonin's tendency to crowd out dopamine if pushed too high. For some (particularly those who have been disabled by crippling anxiety), this is a price they are willing to pay. However for others, this can be almost as bad as anxiety. It will depend on the individual. For example, a complete lack of libido may be viewed differently for a 70 year old man compared to an 18 year old man.

Serotonin is made from dietary l-tryptophan, an amino acid found in a large number of common protein sources. Tryptophan is first converted to 5-htp and then into serotonin. This is why there are supplement products available which contain either of these two steps in the process.

Dopamine (DA)

Dopamine is another incredibly complex neurotransmitter, with vastly different effects depending on where it is acting. It is dopamine which makes drugs like cocaine, amphetamine and heroin addictive, by turning on the reward centres of your brain. However, when you come down from a cocaine or amphetamine high, you get to experience the flip side after the drug has depleted your stores of dopamine. Low on dopamine, you feel a complete lack of motivation, nothing seems interesting, you can't feel pleasure at all and you may be intensely anxious. Low dopamine and low serotonin can both make you anxious, which is why untangling the two is important when looking for the right medication.

A great way of looking at dopamine is that it drives you to do things which your brain views as vital for your survival. Just calling it "the neurotransmitter of pleasure" is too simplistic. If you want to know what dopamine feels like, it is that lovely jolt of pleasure when you think about your favourite food when you are ravenously hungry, or when you think about having sexual intercourse. Dopamine is all about the future. Once you have actually done whatever it was you were looking forward to, dopamine activity drops away. However context is really important here. If the sexual intercourse was with your partner whom you love, after orgasm dopamine falls away to be replaced by the warm, contented glow of serotonin and the bonding hormone oxytocin. However if the sexual intercourse was an impromptu affair with a co-worker (despite you both being married), dopamine can fall away, leaving a hollow feeling of regret. The identical dopamine-driven process happens when you binge on that tub of chocolate chip ice-cream. Dopamine can sometimes drive you to do things you regret.

This issue of context is central to the role of dopamine in mood disorders. Depending on the context, both low dopamine and high dopamine can trigger anxiety. This means that someone could take a dangerously high amount of methamphetamine and trigger a severe panic reaction, only for dopamine to be depleted, whereupon a different flavour of anxiety sets in. This complexity can drive some people to do things which are not in their long-term interests. For example, many amphetamine addicts are actually trying to self-medicate their crippling social anxiety. A socially anxious person who takes meth for the first time will often find that it instantly cures their lifelong inability to interact with groups of people. However unfortunately it is a mirage. Essentially what they are doing is robbing weeks of dopamine to use it all up in a 3 hour concentrated burst. When the meth wears off, their social anxiety will have amplified ten-fold. Then, the next time they try to recapture this wonderful experience of being free of social anxiety, they will need a much higher dose of meth. Both you and I know that this can't end well, however for the person in question, things are not so simple. Meth has the ability to quickly rewire your brain's reward centre, so that it now views the drug as being just as important as food or sex.

The real tragedy here is that there are safe, sustainable ways to gradually boost dopamine without frying your brain with meth.

That said, boosting dopamine comes with its own set of unique challenges. One problem, which it shares with GABA, is that dopamine is notorious for tolerance and addiction. This is the reason why treating mood disorders which are caused by dopaminergic problems can be tricky. In contrast, if you take a serotonergic drug like an SSRI, for the most part [3] you won't need to escalate your dose to maintain the same effect. However, if you took an equivalent drug which boosts dopamine, you will gradually need to increase the dose to get the same effects. There are ways to overcome this problem however they require the guidance of an experienced psychopharmacologist.

This is also an appropriate juncture to address the difference between addiction and dependency, as these are often conflated. There is a major distinction between the two. To illustrate, let's stick with the two previous examples – an SSRI which boosts serotonin and DRI (such as methylphenidate). If you take an SSRI for a few months, you will become physically dependent on it. This means that if it is suddenly stopped, you will experience a range of nasty effects. If you take just about any drug for long enough, your body's inbuilt homeostatic mechanisms will adjust to the drug by changing the density of receptors or the level of neurotransmitter production. So if you then stop suddenly, you will need to gradually adapt – a process which can vary from barely noticeable to incapacitating. This is not addiction. You don't feel compelled to take more of the drug. However, with a dopamine-boosting drug like methylphenidate, if you have addictive tendencies or substance abuse issues, you may feel compelled to take more. This is also caused by a combination of factors such as –

- **Speed of onset and duration of action** – In general, the quicker the drug takes to work and the shorter its half-life, the more addictive it will be. This is why injecting drugs tends to be the quickest path to addiction, as the drug comes on in a euphoric rush. Then, if it doesn't last for long, there can be a sudden, depressing crash which leads to more craving
- **Tolerance** – In an attempt to recapture the initial high, the person continually increases their dose
- **Dopamine-boosting drugs are reinforcing** – Artificially activating your reward centres hijacks your brain. In doing so, this part of your brain decides that the drug is more important than the other stuff that usually activates it, such as sex or food. Eventually, if a dopaminergic drug is abused over a period of time, it desensitises the reward pathway to the point where nothing except the drug is able to activate it. So for someone addicted to meth, cocaine or heroin, obtaining the drug becomes a central feature in their life

---

[3] Occasionally SSRI therapy results in a phenomenon known as "poop out" where the drug inexplicably stops working

When someone stops taking an SSRI, although they will feel pretty darn awful for a while, they won't feel compelled to take the drug. And, in any case, because an SSRI takes so long to work, there is no incentive for the person to restart the drug to make the suffering stop. Chances are that, by the time it starts working again, the most difficult period would have passed. I should point out that there is one exception to this which I will cover later in the book.

Addiction is pathological, damaging to both the addict and those around them. An addict will make the acquisition of the drug the primary goal of each day, then once they obtain the drug, they will have little control over how much they take. Dependency on the other hand, is a normal part of taking any medication long enough for your brain to implement compensatory mechanisms.

Whereas serotonin is synthesised from l-tryptophan, dopamine is made from l-tyrosine. In terms of supplements available, you can also buy supplements containing each step of the dopamine synthesis pathway – l-tyrosine, DL phenylalanine and L-DOPA. One distinction however, is that pure L-DOPA is a powerful pharmaceutical used in the treatment of Parkinson's disease, although you can obtain it via an Indian herb called mucuna pruriens, which is rich in L-DOPA.

Noradrenaline (Norepinephrine, NE)

NE is the close cousin of dopamine and is responsible for a whole host of effects such as its chief role in giving us energy and controlling our circadian rhythm. A malfunctioning NE system is a major contributor to mood disorders, as the physical and psychological sensation of anxiety involves NE and depression is associated with low NE. For example, a central feature of panic disorder is a sudden and powerful activation of the fight or flight system which is caused by a flood of NE being released.

Using this simplified understanding of NE, people sometimes think that they simply need to reduce NE to treat anxiety or to increase it to treat depression. Unfortunately, like dopamine, things are not so simple. For example, drugs like SNRIs and tricyclics (TCAs) often boost NE levels yet can be powerful anti-anxiety agents. It all depends on context and where in the brain the NE is released. This touches on the central principle of my public speaking book, The Excitement Principle. The physical symptoms of anxiety you may experience before giving a presentation to a large group of people are often fairly similar to the excitement you feel before something positive or important is about to happen (Like, for example, when you think your partner is about to propose to you). The key difference is how you view these events.

NE is like the salt you add to a bland dish, accentuating whatever the situation you are in. If you won the lottery and you lacked the ability to produce NE, you will not be able to feel the visceral excitement which enhances the mental feeling of happiness. Sure, you would be happy, but you wouldn't *feel* excited.

As you will soon see, NE plays a key role in the treatment of mood disorders and fortunately there are a range of direct and indirect ways we can modulate NE to modulate mood.

Just the tip of the iceberg

GABA, glutamate, serotonin, dopamine and noradrenaline are the major players in the treatment of mood disorders, however there are countless others which also play a role. Recently, researchers have been studying the endocannabinoid system (which is activated by marijuana) and have found that by activating its receptors (such as CB1 and CB2) a range of effects are triggered which can provide fast and effective relief from anxiety and depression. Or the neuro-peptide *substance P*, which plays a major role in the perception of pain, stress tolerance and anxiety levels.

As complex as the brain is, there are actually only a handful of ways you can treat mood disorders from a pharmacological perspective. I thought it might be helpful to demystify this process to give you a better understanding of why exactly your psychiatrist has chosen a particular medication or combination of medications.

So first, in general terms, irrespective of which drug we are talking about, the vast majority work by harnessing one or more of the following basic processes.

1. Reuptake inhibition

If a drug is a reuptake inhibitor of serotonin, dopamine or noradrenaline, it inhibits the ability of your brain to reabsorb these neurotransmitters, leading to increased amounts floating around in the gap between each brain cell.

2. Receptor agonism

A receptor agonist activates a particular receptor, functioning as a kind of "imposter". So, for example, a dopamine agonist drug functions in the same way as actual dopamine, so if you lack sufficient dopamine, the agonist drug can help bridge the gap, activating dopamine receptors which have been laying idle. It is also important to point out that the word "agonist" doesn't just refer to drugs. Each neurotransmitter is also an agonist of the same receptors.

3. Receptor antagonism

A receptor antagonist essentially functions in the opposite way to an agonist, blocking the receptor so the usual neurotransmitter which activates it cannot gain access. You may have heard of the drugs used to treat high blood-pressure known as *beta-blockers*. These drugs work by blocking certain adrenal receptors, thereby causing blood pressure to drop.

4. Releasing agents

These drugs work by essentially turning up the "tap" which pumps out a particular neurotransmitter into the synapse. So a serotonin releasing agent causes your brain cells to empty their "serotonin storage tanks".

5. Increasing the building blocks of neurotransmitters

Another addition to the above could be an angle often targeted by supplements, which involves taking the building blocks of certain neurotransmitters to hopefully ramp up production. Some target different stages in the process whereby your brain converts an amino acid into a neurotransmitter. Most commonly –

Serotonin – L-tryptophan, 5-htp

Dopamine & Noradrenaline – L-tyrosine, DL Phenylalanine, DOPA

6. Co-factors in the "neurotransmitter production process"

Finally, you could take a supplement which plays a key role in the above process. So, if I use the analogy of making home-made ice-cream, the above amino acids would be the milk and cream. When you make home-made ice-cream, you will also need ingredients such as eggs, or the process won't work properly. In your brain, this process requires certain vitamins and enzymes which are sometimes referred to as *co-factors*. The perfect example of this is a form of folate (vitamin B9) known as l-methylfolate (or Levomefolic acid). The background to folate, why it is so important for sufferers of anxiety and how common it is for people to have issues with it, is so important that I want to spend a few moments explaining.

Firstly, a common question I am asked is what the difference is between folate and folic acid. Essentially, folate is the form found in nature and folic acid is a synthetic form used in supplements or to fortify certain grain-based foods like bread. Why is this distinction important? In answering this, I originally wrote almost two pages in the first draft of this guide, however then decided that these were two of the most boring pages ever written. So I have endeavoured to create a pared back answer to keep things (relatively) snappy. Whenever I need to force myself to be more circumscribed, I revert to dot points, which is what I will do now –

- L-methylfolate is a vital co-factor in the synthesis of serotonin and dopamine. A *co-factor* in this context is something required for the process of creating these neurotransmitters in order to work properly. Think back to one of those classic high-school chemistry class experiments. You would add two ingredients together and nothing would happen until the third was added and then, boom!
- While your body processes folic acid and folate slightly differently, both need to be converted into l-methylfolate before they are useful in this process of creating neurotransmitters
- A fairly large subset of the population has a genetic mutation which prevents them from converting folate and folic acid to l-methylfolate. These people lack a gene known as MTHFR, which normally enables the creation of an enzyme of the same name. You are no doubt wondering what MTHFR stands for right? It stands for *methylenetetrahydrofolate reductase*. I bet you regret asking now.

- The process of converting folate into l-methylfolate is known as the *methylation cycle* and is vital to a huge number of biochemical processes in your body.

To give you a sense of just how important this is for the production of serotonin, variants of l-methylfolate such as Deplin or Metafolin are actually available as a prescription drug to be taken with SSRIs. The reason for this is if you are one of the many people who lack the MTHFR gene, no matter how much you try to boost serotonin with an SSRI, nothing happens because this key ingredient is missing.

If you suspect you may fit into this group, there is an easy genetic test you can have done which will give you the answer. Alternatively, you could just supplement l-methylfolate or take the prescription form. In addition to the reason just mentioned, there is another compelling reason to supplement l-methylfolate instead of folic acid. Some people have an impaired ability to metabolise folic acid, which can lead to elevated levels in the blood, which in turn is associated with a range of negative health consequences.

One final point if you are intending on starting supplementation of an "active" form of folate such as l-methylfolate. There are a range of products on the market which, although there may be slight differences, for your purposes should be considered equivalent. The main examples of these are L-5-MTHFR and folinic acid.

The daunting thing is that folic acid is just the tip. In order to synthesise neurotransmitters, you require sufficient supplies of vitamins and minerals such as magnesium, vitamin c and just about all of the various B-group vitamins (particularly B6 for serotonin synthesis). This is why I always recommend you take a strong, broad spectrum Mega-B product which contains everything in this group. There are also certain multi-B-group products which contain not only the B-group vitamins, but all the other various co-factors for making neurotransmitters. Often these are marketed for people who are "stressed", as stress drains B-group levels as they are all exhausted making serotonin and dopamine.

This highlights just how complex this aspect of brain function is and why often the only option for a psychiatrist is to make an educated guess based on symptoms. And this is probably better than 95% of most cases, where you are handed an SSRI without any particular reference to your symptoms. This is also why I caution people to accept that sometimes you only reach your ideal drug regime through trial and error. To give you an idea, let's use the relationship of anxiety and serotonin as an example. First, your psychiatrist needs to be able to ascertain (with some degree of confidence) that your anxiety is indeed related to problems with serotonin. Even this is not guaranteed, with low dopamine or high noradrenaline having many features which overlap with low serotonin. So let's just assume that your doctor is correct and serotonin is indeed your problem. Next they need to work out what aspect of serotonin function is causing you issues with anxiety. Here are some of the potential causes –

- Insufficient dietary l-tryptophan (lack of building blocks)
- Poor conversion of l-tryptophan to 5-htp
- Poor conversion of 5-htp to serotonin
- Lack of dietary folate needed for the above conversion
- Poor conversion of folate/folic acid to l-methylfolate
- Lack of other co-factors such as magnesium or B6
- Too much dietary l-tyrosine (l-tyrosine can compete with l-tryptophan to cross the blood brain barrier as both require a kind of "shuttle bus" called the large amino acid transporter – this "bus" has limited seats)
- Too much dopamine (this can suppress serotonin functioning)
- Insufficient serotonin release
- Hyperfunctioning serotonin reuptake removing it too quickly from the synapse
- Hyperfunctioning monoamine oxidase is breaking serotonin down too quickly
- Mismatch between serotonin in the synapse and density of serotonin receptors

This is just a selection and this focuses purely on serotonin, so you can easily see the challenge facing doctors. This is also what frustrates me when I see people advocating a "magic bullet" for depression. For example, I have seen many people promoting the supplement 5-htp as a universal panacea for depression. If you lack dietary l-tryptophan or if you are a poor converter, 5-htp could indeed be just what you need. However for most people, the building blocks are not their "rate limiting step", so 5-htp will be ineffective. It takes more personalised care to come up with the solution that addresses whatever it is that is causing your anxiety.

Next, I would like to dispel some common misconceptions I encounter when people are considering which drug[4] would be most effective.

1. **"Drug X worked for my best friend so I want to try that one"**

Everyone is different, with slightly differing genetics, neurochemistry and metabolism. There is no single best drug to treat mood disorders. To confirm this, just visit the 'reviews' page of a site with information on particular drugs. One person says a particular drug was a miracle cure, others say it did nothing and others say it was the worst thing they ever took. For many people SSRIs will be extremely helpful. However even within that single class there are many options and each person responds differently. And this only encompasses those where serotonin is the issue. If you have anxiety or depression due to a different neurotransmitter issue, SSRIs could be counterproductive. This is why the guidance of an experienced expert is vital.

2. **"I don't need to do any research because my doctor will know the best medication for me"**

Sometimes this is true; however we live in an imperfect world. Often doctors are rushed for time and do not have the time to spend several hours with you getting a detailed explanation of your symptoms. They also often don't have time to keep up with the latest research; particularly if you are just visiting a general practitioner (clinical psychologists however will generally be more up to date on research). Your GP has to be a *jack of all trades*, knowing just enough about the most common ailments and enough to be able to then send you to a specialist if you have a more challenging condition.

Also, doctors are, by necessity, naturally risk averse when it comes to treatments. This is one of the most common misconceptions. Your doctor will always take the low-risk option and look for the treatment which is commonly accepted as the safest or most conservative. If your doctor sticks to mainstream, common practices, they do not expose themselves to risk of litigation. For example, if a doctor prescribes the most common SSRI to someone and they then commit suicide, the doctor will not come under additional scrutiny. However, the same doctor tries something novel, new or *off-label* (meaning they prescribe a drug originally developed for another condition) and then their patient commits suicide, they are exposing themselves to the risk of being sued. This is one of the reasons why statins continue to be heavily prescribed, despite a lack of evidence for benefit except in the most severe cases of

---

[4] Anything which decreases anxiety is called *anxiolytic*. Anything which increases anxiety is *anxiogenic*.

hypercholesterolemia or pre-existing heart disease. Due to clever marketing by the makers of statins, if you have elevated cholesterol, the base case for doctors is to recommend statins. If your doctor tells you to get off statins and then you have a heart attack (statistically this WILL happen to someone, irrespective of how unlikely), your doctor could potentially be sued.

3. *"I will stay on my medication for a few months and then stop as soon as I feel better"*

The brain takes a long time to change itself, especially when repairing a lifetime of maladaptive thinking, unhealthy behaviours and off-kilter neurochemistry. For example, meaningful changes to the number and efficiency of serotonin receptors takes a minimum three months (which happens to coincide with the time when your medication should start being in full effect). Medications like SSRIs are like "training wheels" which keep you from falling while you learn new behaviours and ways of thinking. If you take your training wheels off too soon, you risk crashing your "mental bicycle". In general you should be prepared to be on the medication for a minimum of one year, and more if your doctor deems it appropriate. Some people only need drugs for a year or so before they are able to stop, while others will need to take something indefinitely. Please ensure you make an informed decision in consultation with an expert, making sure that you continue or stop for the right reasons. Too many times I have seen people stop taking their medication for the wrong reasons, only to undo a year or more of progress.

If treating mood disorders simply involved boosting serotonin, you would be "cured" within a few days, as this is how long it takes for SSRIs to increase levels of serotonin. However we are only beginning to scratch the surface of the exact mechanisms which underlie mood disorders. Some researchers now believe that SSRIs treat mood disorders for reasons unrelated to the increase in serotonin. Psychotropic medications are long term healers, however you must give it time to let your brain regrow. Also at the cognitive or behavioural level, you need to give it time to let new, more positive thought and behaviour patterns to take hold and for the old, pathological habits to be extinguished properly.

4. *"I tried an SSRI for a week or so but it was terrible so I stopped"*

This is the most disturbing comment you see everywhere on internet forums and in drug reviews on the internet. Many doctors do not explain this most vital of points – when you start a new medication (particularly SSRIs), you will likely feel *worse* initially. The confusing thing is that these initial symptoms perfectly mimic your anxiety or depression worsening. You need to prepare to feel worse initially and plan your life around this period accordingly. The encouraging thing is that many people attest that the best medication they tried was the one that made them feel the worst at the start. Here is a good way of thinking about it – if it is worsening your symptoms, you know that the medication is targeting the part of your brain or the particular neurochemical which is causing you issues.

However, this is also where some care and judgement are required. You need to give the medication enough time to work, however if a) you have not improved after 3-4 weeks or b) you are finding the effects (or side effects) unbearable, return to your doctor to discuss alternatives. Often a change to a similar medication in the same class can make all the difference.

5. *"I heard that antidepressants are no better than placebos and that drug companies lie and cheat to make them look effective"*

Actually, this is, strictly speaking, half-true. Yes, drug companies lie and cheat, as evidenced by the reboxetine debacle which you will read about later in the book. In a review by Dr Ben Goldacre (*senior clinical research fellow and well-known author of Bad Science*) and Professor Carl Heneghan (*professor of evidence based medicine, Centre for Evidence-Based Medicine, University of Oxford*), published in the *British Medical Journal* (BMJ), this very topic was addressed head-on. Among other things, it was point out that –

- 97% of all trials paid for by drug companies found that (surprise, surprise) the drug belonging to the company who paid for the trial was found to be superior. Yes, this is as awful as it sounds.
- Trial results were distorted by commercial factors such as incentives paid to doctors. An example given was where a drug company would incentivise doctors to select certain patients who would be conducive to achieving a favourable result.

This, in addition to the reboxetine fiasco, makes for sobering reading. However there is a silver lining.

Firstly, the BMJ study on reboxetine clearly demonstrated something which was lost in the hue & cry. Whilst it clearly showed that reboxetine is no better than placebo, it also showed that SSRIs are more effective than both reboxetine and placebo. The general theme of those opposed to SSRIs is that they are no better than placebo and when they are better than placebo, it is because the drug company fudged the numbers. However the BMJ study used all available data where reboxetine was compared to SSRIs and placebo with the express purpose of uncovering the truth by removing selection bias from the equation. This comprehensive study debunked a common myth which has surrounded SSRIs for the past decade or more.

The BMJ study also weakened another argument used by some anti-antidepressant[5] types such as Irving Kirsch (author of the book *The Emperor's New Drugs: Exploding*

---

[5] Or should that double-negative be changed to "pro-depressant"? No, that doesn't sound right.

the Anti-depressant Myth). Kirsch, who conducted his own study a while back, reached the conclusion that antidepressants only work better than placebo because the drugs themselves create a different kind of placebo effect which is caused by their side-effects. Kirsch's hypothesis is that, when a patient takes an antidepressant, they start to experience side-effects (both unpleasant and neutral), which creates a subtle message in their mind that "the drug must be working, because I can feel its effects". They then draw a simple conclusion that the side-effects are a sign that the drug is working, so they then start to improve due to placebo effect.

Don't get me wrong. I think this is no doubt a factor. I have even had someone tell me that when they started taking escitalopram (Lexapro), they started getting strange tingling sensations which seemed to run along their scalp. They interpreted this sensation with optimism and their mood started improving.

However to say that this is accurate in all (or even most) cases would be drawing quite a long bow. The BMJ review demonstrates this because they found that reboxetine was associated with the most side-effects, yet was the least effective drug. When patients start taking reboxetine and start feeling like they have just overdosed on some cheap and nasty pseudoephedrine-based cold & flu medication, according to Kirsch's hypothesis they should then start feeling better due to placebo. However if anything, the opposite is true in most cases.

A key factor would be the type of side-effect. Tingling sensations in your scalp is one thing, however nausea, diarrhoea and agitation is another. I know of many patients for whom the side-effects were a source of immense disappointment.

When we strip away all of the vested interests and simplistic models, we are left with our best understanding of the truth (as it stands today) –

1. A little more than half the population will be adequately treated by the first drug they try
2. The figures are even worse for mild-to-moderate depression, where there is a lack of compelling evidence supporting the use of drugs
3. However, after trial and error, most people find a drug (or combination of drugs) which works for them
4. A tiny number of people never benefit from any drug
5. Your "perfect drug" and the perfect drug for your friend or partner are unlikely to be the same

And each time new evidence arises which contradicts any of the above, we must have the intellectual courage and cognitive flexibility to adjust our views.

Do you even need to take drugs in the first place?

Firstly, please consult your doctor or health professional regarding this. Please do not take information you obtain on the internet or read in an eBook as fact.

However, to enable you to at least form a well-considered position on this crucial point, here are some questions you have to ask yourself first –

- *Am I just depressed or anxious due to a specific, isolated event?* As you have made it this far reading a book on psychotropic medications, I doubt this would be the case for you. However it is worth making the point that occasional, time-limited anxiety or depression is normal and doesn't signify a mood disorder and *certainly* doesn't warrant medication, unless it is needed to help you sleep for a short while.

- *Do I have any physical symptoms which aren't going away?* Mood disorders are associated with a surprising array of physical symptoms. It is incredibly common for someone to visit their doctor due to what seem to be signs of a serious neurological condition such as multiple sclerosis, only to learn that anxiety or depression is the culprit. Some of the more common ones include sleeping problems (insomnia, poor quality sleep etc.), stomach aches, headaches and tremors. If your mood problems are beginning to manifest in symptoms like these, it can sometimes be a good indicator that medication could be helpful.

- *Do I feel suicidal or like I can't cope?* If you are experiencing suicidal ideation (thinking about suicide), see your doctor immediately. They will be able to provide pharmaceutical support and refer you to a specialist, where you will most likely receive priority attention. If you are in immediate danger, please either reach out to a family member or friend to provide urgent support. Also remember that in many countries there will be a special phone number you can call if you are in desperate straits, where a kind, sensitive expert will be able to help.

Medications for anxiety and depression can be extremely unpleasant to come off and withdraw from. You have to bear this in mind before deciding to start taking them. Some people have said that they are worse than heroin to withdraw from! That said, fear of the withdrawal process should never dictate whether you decide to start anxiolytics. It should be something you bear in mind, along with a range of other factors, when deciding whether your situation is serious enough to warrant going doing the medication path. To decide against starting a drug that could stop you from feeling terrible, because you may or may not feel bad for a while when stopping, is not sensible. Getting better should be your number one concern. The question is whether you or your specialist feel you could get better without the help of medication.

Dosage

You may need to do some experimentation regarding the right dosage for you. The difference between success and failure is often down to the dosage. As an example, there are some drugs which affect different neurotransmitters, depending on the dosage. Venlafaxine is an example of this. At low dosages, venlafaxine only affects serotonin, while at higher dosages it also affects noradrenaline (norepinephrine).

Unless otherwise instructed by your psychiatrist, always start low and titrate (increase) up until you find a dosage that works for you. This is important for two reasons. Firstly, you can avoid most of the unpleasant start-up effects by starting slowly and working your way up, allowing your brain to get used to the drug. Secondly, you should always try to work out the best dosage for yourself and try to avoid going over this dosage. The lower you can keep your dosage, the more chance you have of avoiding side-effects or unpleasant withdrawal symptoms. However you also need to bear in mind that there is a minimum therapeutic dose for each medication and you need to ensure you are over this level, otherwise you may be defeating the purpose of taking them in the first place.

Antidepressants are not "happy pills"

As mentioned previously, the best way to think of medication is as *training wheels for your brain*. Antidepressants keep your emotions in a narrower range (both up *and* down). The upside to this is obvious but the downside is you are unlikely to feel 'highs' as intensely as when you are not on them. Some people refer to this as *blunted emotions*. I have generally found the 'training wheels' analogy to be helpful for those I work with, because with training wheels you are not going to be able to go as fast as you would with two wheels, but you won't fall over and hurt yourself!

Get comfortable - you will probably have to stay on them for a while

If you decide to take a medication for anxiety or depression, you should consider a minimum of six to twelve months to gain full therapeutic effect. Antidepressants don't just suddenly increase the level of serotonin in your brain, causing you to immediately feel better. You need to allow enough time for neuroplastic change to occur. In his book on depression, The Noonday Demon, author Andrew Solomon indicated that some experts believe that if you have long term issues with depression or anxiety, you should consider indefinite treatment. These specialists hypothesize that coming on and off antidepressants multiple times can cause lasting negative changes in certain parts of the brain. The general rule of thumb is that you should consider one year to be the minimum time to stay on antidepressants. Let me stress this again – *one of the most common problems with anxiolytic treatment is where people stop as soon as they start feeling better*. This will almost always result in an immediate relapse. Promise yourself you will stick it out, even if you are feeling better or consider yourself "cured".

Don't expect the medication to do all the work

I always warn against the idea of going on medication, only to then sit back and wait for the drug to do all the work. You have to work on yourself at the same time, otherwise when you stop taking them you will just revert back to your old habits. Change your thinking and your lifestyle to be more conducive to mental wellbeing.

Should I stay on some form of medication indefinitely?

This is a complicated topic also, however in general I don't believe most depressed or anxious people have a natural, inbuilt chemical imbalance which causes their issues. I think there is a complicated cause and effect loop between thoughts and neurochemistry. That is, I tend to think that low levels of neurotransmitters like serotonin is more of an *effect* of depression rather than a *cause*. However they are interrelated, which is why modulating one can affect the other, meaning, you can change your thinking to increase serotonin and you can increase serotonin (through drugs) to change your thinking.

For a variety of reasons, some people decide to stay on medication for good. I personally have several friends who say that they "prefer themselves" on medication rather than off. This is a personal decision and you should not judge yourself negatively if you decide to stay on your medication for good. Coming off your medication can be extremely challenging, so you shouldn't beat yourself up if you don't feel up to it. There are two decisions here, not one. First you need to establish whether you are ready to stop. This should always be done in consultation with your doctor or psychiatrist. Secondly, if the decision is made to stop, you need to choose the best time to do so. Never withdraw from medications during major life events, when you are stressed or when you have significant commitments at work or at home.

Suicide risk when starting antidepressants

As you may have read, starting antidepressants is occasionally associated with increased suicidal ideation. This is quite rare, so for most people it is unlikely that starting your medication will make you feel suicidal. However, if you do find that you are having thoughts of suicide or self-harm, you need to contact a professional (preferably your doctor) immediately. The commonly accepted theory is that starting antidepressants can give you an initial burst of energy before they actually start improving your mood. It is common for someone with an anxiety disorder to also have co-existing depression, so there is a chance that someone can start medication while both depressed and anxious. In rare cases, the medication can act like a "jump start", giving them the energy to follow through and act on their thoughts of self-harm. However it is important to point out that this is usually limited to drugs which act on serotonin, such as SSRIs or tricyclics, not pure anxiolytics like benzodiazepines.

While it is not common to feel suicidal when starting medication, it is quite common however for your depression or anxiety to briefly worsen during this start-up period. Again, there are a few theories as to why this is the case. The strongest theory is that, while your brain is adjusting to the drug, it initially senses too much serotonin floating around in the synapse (because the drug has started keeping serotonin levels higher than before) and consequently, throttles back how much serotonin is created, leading to a temporary deficit. There are a type of receptor for serotonin called *autoreceptors* which sense levels of serotonin in the synapse and make adjustments accordingly. I have seen these autoreceptors referred to as "air traffic controllers" at the airport. When you start an SSRI, these autoreceptors appear to throttle back the amount of serotonin released into the synapse. It takes a while for this whole system to eventually find homeostatis and you start feeling better.

The theory itself is not important. What is important however is that often, feeling worse initially is a good sign that the drug is working. In layman's terms, if you are taking a drug to treat anxiety and your anxiety worsens initially, it is often a sign that the drug is working in exactly the right place. However, you need to bear in mind that the difference between start-up problems and having the wrong drug for your particular brain can be subtle. This is why all this should be done with the input of an expert.

Side effects

In general, each drug and each class of drug has a range of different side-effects, however the most common side-effects associated with these drugs are weight gain (or weight *loss* sometimes), sexual dysfunction (lack of libido, problems achieving an erection or problem achieving orgasm), blunted emotions (lack of emotional highs and lows), agitation (or somnolence). It is important to note that side-effects tend to increase as the dosage increases.

Each class of medication has different side-effects, so this can sometimes dictate which treatment will be best for you. For example, SSRIs are known for sexual side-effects whereas tricyclic drugs are known for *anticholinergic* problems such as dry mouth and constipation. However I should point out that if you are on a small to average dose, even if you do experience side-effects to begin with, they should gradually settle down and resolve.

If you continue to experience troubling side-effects you can discuss this with your doctor who may either switch you to another medication or add an additional medication to deal with the side-effects. Many people are opposed to this in principle as they worry about becoming trapped on a never-ending merry-go-round of drugs. Naturally, if you are taking three or four different drugs to deal with side-effects it can be a bit like playing "whack-a-mole", however adding a single additional drug to your primary antidepressant can be very effective. For example, by adding mirtazapine to an SSRI, you can treat both the sexual side-effects and sleep disturbance, not to mention getting a small mood boost or a reduction in anxiety well.

Weight gain would be near the top of the most common side-effects of the antidepressant-style drugs. Some experienced psychiatrists I deal with have indicated that weight gain while on SSRI therapy is highly understated in the official clinical trial material and most definitely understated in drug company marketing materials. Some supporting trial data for common SSRIs can indicate that weight gain on the SSRI in question is not statistically significant. However in real world examples, mean weight gain on SSRIs has been estimated as high as 20lb. This is significantly higher in the case of mirtazapine and another order of magnitude higher if you are also augmented with an anti-psychotic such as olanzapine or quetiapine.

As I often tell people, depression is not just a simple case of "neurotransmitter imbalance" or a "lack of serotonin". This is evidenced by the fact that there are a huge number of drugs which can treat depression or anxiety - many of which have mechanisms of action which share no similarities at all.

It is also important to point out that, in many cases, when a drug works, it's not necessarily because of its primary action. For example, as mentioned previously, some researchers believe that SSRIs work for reasons wholly independent of their serotonergic effects. Whether it is due to their action in boosting levels of BDNF (brain-derived neurotrophic factor – a kind of "fertilizer" for your brain), or because they decrease neural inflammation, the key point is whether they work or not. This is one point which frustrates me immensely when I read poorly-informed attacks on antidepressants. Anti-drug types will try to pick apart the entire *serotonin theory of depression*, giving the impression that this proves that SSRIs don't work. The idea that an imbalance of serotonin causes anxiety and depression may ultimately be proven incorrect. In fact, personally I think it is indeed wrong (or at least, a gross simplification). However this doesn't have any bearing on whether these drugs are effective, as we are slowly discovering new things they do inside our brains.

In the vast majority of cases, it is more than likely that your doctor will start with an SSRI. This is because they are safe, effective and are widely used, giving them confidence in terms of risks and benefits. In many cases, this will be the right choice, however for others, a non-SSRI option would be more effective. Even within the SSRI class, many people who don't respond to the first one, respond to subsequent alternative SSRIs. Your doctor or specialist may however also add in fast acting anxiolytic like a benzodiazepine for the start-up period, as SSRIs can take a while to start working and can increase anxiety for a few days.

In fact, one of the chief reasons I dedicated an entire guide to medications for anxiety and depression was because I was seeing so many people who tried a single SSRI and it didn't help them. These people then just settle for a sub-optimal treatment option or give up altogether. The key point is that there are a huge number of options, across many different classes of drugs. Unfortunately, many GPs are unaware of these alternatives, having no experience outside the standard, common options. Quite often, the perfect drug for you may be a left-field, off-label option. Or it may be a recently released drug. There is a huge time lag between a particular drug becoming available to when your doctor will feel comfortable prescribing it. Again this is where a specialist psychiatrist has a huge advantage, as they are aware of every possible medication and are typically more comfortable trying "adventurous" options when all else has failed.

If there is one piece of advice I can give which I have given to countless others – sometimes with "life-changing" effects, it would be -

Don't give up and don't settle for "near enough is good enough". Think about it this way – Say there are 20 different medications commonly used to treat anxiety and depression. Even with a great psychiatrist and excellent diagnosis, the probability that you will find your "perfect" (or perhaps a better way of putting it would be – "best for you") drug the first time is quite low. If you are not happy with how you have responded to a particular drug, or the side-effects you are experiencing, don't hesitate to return to your psychiatrist to discuss alternatives. It won't have been a wasted experience either. How you respond to the first medication can tell your doctor a lot, helping them to work out whether you simply need a dosage adjustment or whether a different drug is warranted. Many times have I seen someone about to give up, only to stumble on the option that ends up working for them.

Drugs by category

As many drugs have multiple mechanisms of action, categorising them becomes somewhat arbitrary, however I have broken them up into what I feel is the clearest way possible, based on their mechanism of action. In the vast majority of cases, your doctor or psychiatrist will want to start with either an SSRI or an SNRI as the "first-line" option. Many will also routinely provide a script for a benzodiazepine as a short-term option for mitigating start-up anxiety which can be a common problems. This is especially the case for those starting the SSRI for an anxiety disorder or those suffering from anxious depression. If the first SSRI doesn't work, the doctor may then either try another SSRI or another class altogether.

As an SSRI forms at least part of the treatment for the vast majority of cases, I will spend more time discussing them, compared to MAOIs, which are only typically used in rare cases these days.

SSRIs are usually the first line of treatment for most cases of anxiety or depression for several main reasons. Firstly, they have the safest overdose profile, which means that they are close to impossible to overdose on. This contrasts with drugs like TCAs (*tricyclic antidepressants*) or benzodiazepines like Xanax (alprazolam) which are easier to overdose on, whether deliberately or inadvertently. It is worth remembering that in the back of any psychiatrist's mind, they will be assessing their patient to establish whether there is any suicide risk. Consequently they will usually be cautious in terms of avoiding drugs which could enable this. Secondly, SSRIs have a relatively mild side-effect profile compared to other medications. Whilst some people find the side-effects intolerable, compared to older drugs, most people find SSRI side-effects to be transient in nature, quickly fading as the patient adjusts. However for some people, these side-effects can be intensely unpleasant and remain an issue beyond the initial start-up period.

Those of us lucky enough to be born in this era of second and third-generation antidepressants usually don't realise just how difficult the old-school drugs really were for patients (which unfortunately can be cold comfort if you are experiencing troubling side-effects from an SSRI).

Finally, another rarely reported reason for their use as first-line antidepressants and anxiolytics is that they are the accepted mainstream treatment. If you visit your doctor and they start you on SSRIs, whereupon you have a bad reaction or self-harm, they are relatively protected from a legal perspective, as they are simply conforming to the mainstream accepted treatment protocol. Put another way, if your doctor puts you on a new type of medication or one which is not usually used to treat mood disorders and something bad happens, they are exposing themselves to questions being asked and even possible litigation.

However, importantly, according to some experts, SSRIs can be inferior to TCAs or MAOIs in cases of moderate to severe anxiety and depression, but tend to be safer and have a milder side-effect profile. Treating mood disorders doesn't begin and end with SSRIs, so if you see no benefit from them after giving them a decent trial, don't feel dispirited, as there are many more options available.

How do they work?

If you were able to look into a super-powerful, high-resolution microscope (many times more powerful than what we have today) and could see your brain at the cellular level, to the degree that you could see two individual brain cells, you would see something interesting. These two neurons would use neurotransmitters like serotonin and dopamine to communicate with one another across the gap between them (this gap is known as a *synapse*). The first neuron would release a neurotransmitter which would float across to the second neuron, fit into the right receptor (like a lock to the neurotransmitter's key) and the message would be sent. It is important to point out that this is a massively simplified representation for the purposes of this topic. In reality there are countless neurotransmitters floating around in the synapse, with huge numbers of each individual type. Now, if we look specifically at serotonin, there is also a *transporter molecule* known as *SERT*, whose job it is to mop up any serotonin floating around in the synapse and take it back to the first neuron for breakdown and recycling. This process is known as *reuptake*.

The *serotonin theory of depression* states that in people with anxiety and depression, there is insufficient serotonin floating around, decreasing the probability that certain messages will be passed from neuron to neuron. SSRIs work by inhibiting the reuptake of serotonin by blocking the action of SERT, the transporter molecule. By blocking this process of removing serotonin, levels of this neurotransmitter gradually increase. If you have anxiety or depression associated with low levels of serotonin, this should gradually start making you feel less anxious or depressed. The word "if" is important here. Despite what you may have read or been told, not all anxiety or depression is caused by low serotonin. There are a huge number of factors at play here. In your case, it may be another neurotransmitter altogether which is responsible for your anxiety. Or it may be another neurological process. Or the reason may even lie outside of your brain, with a stressful life situation or another environmental factor. And even if serotonin was the source of your problems, we still couldn't say with certainty that your anxiety or depression is caused by low serotonin.

To give you an idea of the complexity we face in terms of understanding the causes of anxiety disorders, many researchers believe that SSRIs treat anxiety for reasons unrelated to serotonin, something that shocks most people I talk to. There are many factors at work which could be behind the reason why SSRIs are effective. For example, they increase the amount of BDNF (*brain-derived neurotrophic factor*) in your brain. BDNF is a kind of "fertilizer" for brain cells, enabling your brain to repair and regenerate. SSRIs also possess powerful anti-inflammatory properties, potentially reducing neural inflammation, which is another possible cause of anxiety and depression.

These alternate models of depression (and therefore, by extension, hypotheses for why SSRIs work) are important for giving you a more holistic understanding of your brain, potentially leading you towards more targeted therapies. So let's briefly look at some of these factors in more detail.

Boosting BDNF to drive neuroplasticity

Some research has shown that SSRIs increase certain *plastic* changes in the brain, helping you to grow new neurons and connections between these neurons. Research suggests that this process is underpinned by BDNF. One thing I find interesting is that another way you can boost levels of BDNF is by engaging in cardiovascular exercise and weight training – both of which are effective treatments for mood disorders in themselves. This is one of the reasons why I wrote an entire guide on this topic, as it is one of the most exciting new areas of research into anxiety and depression.

This process of SSRIs triggering growth in the brain is a potential reason behind why SSRIs take up to three months to become effective (as plastic brain changes are believed to take around this period of time). Tests have shown that blood concentrations of serotonin peak after three days of SSRI therapy, so the increase in serotonin alone appears to be only partially linked to the efficacy of SSRIs.

Suppressing REM sleep

Recent research has linked abnormally high levels of REM sleep with mood disorders and in particular, major depression. Therefore, the fact that SSRIs suppress REM sleep may be another reason for their efficacy. My personal opinion is that one of the primary purposes of REM sleep is to help our brain process highly emotional issues, and in particular, those which remain unresolved. If this is the case, it therefore makes sense that when you are going through an emotional or stressful period you will have more REM sleep. In my case, if I have a night of what seems like lots of REM sleep, I always wake up feeling unrefreshed. One of the main problems with having too much REM sleep is that often it comes at the expense of deep, *slow wave* sleep, which is when your brain conducts its most crucial repair and restoration work. Notably, it is believed that this is when the replenishment of neurotransmitters goes into overdrive.

Cooling down neural inflammation

Recent research has shown that anxiety and depression are often associated with abnormally high levels of inflammation. It remains unclear as to whether this is a cause or effect of the underlying illness; however SSRIs modulate the effects of pro-inflammatory substances in the body called *cytokines*. Many researchers now believe that inflammation could be the culprit in certain mood disorders and are therefore developing medications which target the inflammatory process. If I were to put on my "evolutionary psychology hat" for a moment, I think the link between anxiety and inflammation makes perfect sense. When we experience fear, it sets off a cascade of hormonal and neurochemical reactions which are all directed towards fighting, fleeing and then, if you don't get eaten, repairing any resultant injuries. Your body makes a wild guess that if something has caused you to feel intensely afraid, there is a strong chance you could suffer a life-threatening injury if the source of this fear attacks you. Your body's inflammatory process is a major component of this, as inflammation is caused by the production of a range of substances which repair damage. So if you are chronically anxious or suffer from regular panic, you may have an inflammatory process which is locked in the "on" position. However you will note that the direction of causation here is unclear. I can certainly see how chronic anxiety would lead to chronic inflammation, however that doesn't tell us the reason for the anxiety in the first place. Clearly more work in this area is required.

You may get worse before you get better

It never fails to amaze me how many people are simply given a prescription for a particular medication without any further explanation regarding what they may experience and how to prepare appropriately. The initial start-up period for SSRIs can be challenging, to the point where some people self-harm. So the key message is *patience*. You may need to grit your teeth and ride out the initial 4-6 weeks before things should then start to improve. Most people start seeing an improvement in 3-4 weeks, however it can take longer in some cases. The secret to getting through the first few weeks is to maintain hope. Sometimes a difficult journey is only made possible by seeing the destination in the distance. However I also acknowledge that the very disorders we are trying to treat are often associated with a lack of hope or an inability to imagine what it would be like to feel happy or calm again. So if hope is absent, some creative visualisation can be incredibly important. This is why I theorise that some patients commit suicide during the SSRI start-up period. If you are unaware of this tendency to initially worsen when starting an SSRI, it would be enormously dispiriting, tragically causing some to essentially give up on life. However, if you understood that this was a temporary thing, summoning the motivation to endure would be much easier.

Which is the best SSRI?

This is perhaps the single most common question asked on depression or anxiety-related internet forums. However it is the equivalent of asking people *"Mac or PC?"*[6]

Despite what you may hear from some, no SSRI is clinically proven to be the "best" for every person, with huge variations in each individual's response. Each SSRI has a slightly different mode of action or is metabolised a different way, so if you don't feel better after a month or so, don't be shy in discussing alternatives with your doctor. Some are more sedating, whereas others are more activating. This means that if you are lacking energy or motivation, an activating SSRI may be useful. Conversely, if you are agitated, anxious or suffering from insomnia, a sedating SSRI may be a better option.

---

[6] Every Mac user reading this analogy will probably dispute this, I should add.

Variations between different SSRIs

Since the FDA approved the first SSRI (Prozac) for the treatment of depression in 1987, numerous variations have subsequently been developed. Despite all having the inhibition of serotonin reuptake as their common trait, there are surprisingly large variations in how they are metabolised or the supplemental actions they have in addition to serotonin reuptake inhibition. This can result in dramatically different responses across patients. An individual SSRI can be life-changing for some and intolerable for others. In this sense, the expertise of a psychiatrist is partially a function of their ability to identify the best option initially, and partially a function of their ability to respond if the first drug doesn't work. In this scenario, knowing whether another SSRI would be appropriate or whether a drug of a different class would be better, can be the difference between a good psychiatrist and a *great* psychiatrist.

So let's now look at each of these individual SSRIs in detail.

Fluoxetine (*Prozac*)

Fluoxetine was the first SSRI developed back in the 1980s, and to this day is probably the most famous, despite the fact that its usage has waned in recent years as newer drugs have become available. This is not necessarily because it is less effective than the newer drugs, however now that it has gone off-patent (the original developer no longer has exclusive marketing rights), it is not promoted to doctors any more.

Fluoxetine still has a valuable role to play in psychopharmacology, as it possess some unique actions not seen in other SSRIs. However the most distinctive aspect of fluoxetine is its extremely long half-life compared to other SSRIs. This means that a single dose can stay in your system for a few days, compared to others which typically only last for 24 hours. Due to this long half-life, fluoxetine is often used as a tapering drug when both doctor and patient agree that it is appropriate to gradually withdraw from SSRI treatment. This is due to the fact that fluoxetine's long half-life gives you a built-in "gentle landing", as the drug leaves your system much more slowly than other SSRIs. In this scenario, you would be switched from your usual SSRI (such as sertraline or escitalopram) to fluoxetine, before you then slowly taper down your dose of fluoxetine.

The other benefit of fluoxetine's long half-life is that if you forget a dose, you are unlikely to notice, as long as you restart it the following day. This is an important consideration for the young, the elderly, or those with memory problems.

Another unique aspect of fluoxetine is that, along with its SSRI action, it also acts as a mild 5-HT receptor antagonist and a σ_1 (sigma-1) receptor agonist, however there is debate around whether these effects are relevant to the drug's efficacy. Large doses of fluoxetine have also been shown to boost dopamine and noradrenaline, however again the meaningfulness of this is unclear. As I have mentioned previously, antagonising certain serotonin receptors can improve symptoms of anxiety and depression.

Like most SSRIs, fluoxetine is associated with increased anxiety during the start-up period. Whilst this anxiety will soon settle down in most cases, your doctor may initially prescribe a low dose benzodiazepine during the early stages to mitigate this anxiety. The good news is that anecdotally, I have found that those who suffer from the biggest spike in anxiety while starting fluoxetine tend to ultimately have a better response to it.

Fluoxetine's long half-life can also be a double-edged sword when dosage adjustments are needed, as there can be a long lag between a change in dose and the results of this change becoming clear. For the same reason, fluoxetine can also take a bit longer before it starts to take effect. For example, whereas other SSRIs take only a few days to reach stable levels in your system, fluoxetine can take anywhere from 4-8 weeks.

Another important aspect of fluoxetine which many doctors fail to account for is its ability to potently inhibit certain cytochrome P450 enzymes, which are needed for the metabolism of a huge number of drugs. For example, fluoxetine can inhibit the conversion of codeine into morphine or the metabolism of beta-blockers such as propranolol. Considering that propranolol is used to treat dangerously high blood pressure, the importance of understanding these fluoxetine interactions becomes clear.

The standard fluoxetine dosage for depression and anxiety disorders is usually 20mg, with most experts recommending you start on 10mg and titrate up gradually. I tend to be more conservative with SSRI starting dosages, as the last thing anyone wants is to have things derailed by an intolerable start-up. I therefore prefer 5mg as a more cautious starting point.

This is also an ideal juncture for me to address the use of SSRIs to treat OCD. In comparison to depression and other anxiety disorders, OCD usually requires significantly higher dosages to be effective. So whereas the typical fluoxetine dosage is 20mg for other mood disorders, OCD treatment can involve dosages as high as 80mg. I tend to think that many people taking SSRIs for depression or generalised anxiety disorder (GAD) are actually on an unnecessarily high dose, whereas often the opposite is true of OCD patients, who tend to be on dosages well short of the level required. Another aspect where OCD differs from the other mood disorders is the treatment response time. OCD can take longer to respond to medication, sometimes requiring as much as 12 weeks before it becomes clear as to whether the drug is working.

If, after an adequate period of time, at an adequately high dosage, your OCD symptoms don't improve, your doctor will then look at switching to an alternative drug. This process also diverges from other mood disorders. If you have depression or another type of anxiety disorder, quite often a different SSRI will be tried as the second options. However with OCD, the standard second-line option is to switch to the tricyclic clomipramine (which I will cover later in the book). Alternatively, there is the option of adding a drug which modulates glutamate activity (which I will also address later).

Just one final point on the treatment of OCD. As you would probably imagine, with OCD requiring high dose SSRI or tricyclic treatment, non-drug therapies like herbals or other supplements will be inadequate in the vast majority of cases. While there are a range of supplements such as St. John's Wort and rhodiola rosea which can be surprisingly effective for mild-to-moderate depression and anxiety, there are no supplements with compelling clinical trial evidence for the treatment of OCD. One that does however show promise as an adjunct to medication is n-acetylcysteine (NAC), due to its anti-glutamatergic effects.

Sertraline *(Zoloft)*

Along with escitalopram, sertraline is currently the first-line SSRI in many cases these days. The reason for sertraline's popularity is not immediately clear, however it is believed to be one of the strongest of the SSRIs in terms of serotonin reuptake (along with paroxetine). If you are in a deep, dark hole, many doctors will reach for sertraline before any other SSRI. Whilst I maintain my view that the response to SSRIs is highly variable across individuals (therefore making any blanket statements around superiority misguided), in the largest meta-analysis of its kind, sertraline and escitalopram were found to be the most effective. However, individual variation, along with the fact that its superiority over other SSRIs was only modest in statistical terms, makes this a relatively unimportant factor. I guess the only useful information we can derive from this analysis is that we know, at the very least, that sertraline is *as* effective as other SSRIs across the general population.

The reason for its effectiveness perhaps lies in its unique action on both serotonin and dopamine. Dopamine is often the forgotten neurotransmitter these days, with the mainstream focus on serotonin as the prime culprit behind depression and anxiety. As mentioned earlier, dopamine is vital for motivation and feelings of pleasure and is therefore, unsurprisingly, the primary neurotransmitter behind the rewarding, and therefore addictive, properties of recreational drugs such as cocaine and methamphetamine. By increasing levels of dopamine (which is what sertraline does, albeit modestly), sertraline can often give you a boost in motivation and restore your ability to feel pleasure doing activities that interest you. However it is also important to point out that sertraline boosts dopamine only modestly, in an unusual way, in a certain part of the brain. If you take a drug which simply boosts dopamine all over the place (particularly in your reward centres, like the nucleus accumbens or the VTA), it will feel distinctly pleasurable. However sertraline doesn't do this. In both animal models and human trials, sertraline is not reinforcing like other dopaminergic drugs. For many people I have worked with, they have indicated that they didn't feel much of a dopamine "kick", however this could be a factor of both dopaminergic potency and its long half-life. As I have mentioned elsewhere in this book, one of the key drivers behind a drug's addictiveness is how quickly it comes on after administration. Sertraline take hours to reach maximum plasma concentration, perhaps creating a long enough lag that it loses its rewarding properties.

Sertraline's effects on dopamine reuptake are sixty-times less potent than its serotonin reuptake properties, so I think it would be inadvisable to focus on sertraline for its dopamine enhancing properties alone. However for some people, this "bonus extra" could be a defining component of your response to sertraline compared to more serotonin-focused SSRIs.

In addition, sertraline also possesses a modest ability to boost levels of noradrenaline. In combination with its potent action on serotonin and an ability to give dopamine a slight boost, sertraline is known as one of the most activating SSRIs. This is important for several reasons. Firstly, it is associated with the side-effects you would expect of a stimulating drug, such as a tendency to exacerbate insomnia during start-up. More importantly however, its stimulating properties tend to make it more suitable for lethargic depression states and less suitable for anxious depression. However interestingly, after chronic treatment, sertraline can be an effective option for anxiety disorders, as long as you can endure an initial worsening of anxiety during start-up.

One of the complications here (which is something I will address later in this section) is that dopamine has a wide range of effects throughout the brain. Depending on the type of anxiety, dopamine can either improve things or make them worse. For example, those suffering from social anxiety tend to respond well to drugs which boost dopamine such as dexamphetamine, because dopamine can give people social confidence. However if someone with generalised anxiety disorder took amphetamine of any kind, it could very well trigger a state of intense anxiety. Again, at the risk of sounding like a broken record, this is further reason why the input of an expert is needed.

All SSRIs are associated with various forms of sexual dysfunction (lack of interest, inability to achieve erection or orgasm etc.), and sertraline's potency means it is also no different. However of the SSRIs, sertraline's association with sexual dysfunction is the most unclear. So a better way to express this would be to say that if you matched a dosage of sertraline with an equivalent dosage of escitalopram so that the serotonin effects were identical, sertraline should have less sexual side-effects. There are potentially two main reasons for this. Firstly, sertraline's dopamine reuptake inhibition should at least partially offset the ability of serotonin to kill your libido. Secondly, sertraline appears to have the least prolactin-boosting effect among all SSRIs.

One of the reasons why SSRIs mess with sexual function is they boost a hormone called prolactin, which in turn then suppresses dopamine. Among other functions, prolactin is released immediately following orgasm, causing the refractory period, where the idea of further sexual activity becomes unappealing. Our caveman brains want us to stick around and look after the baby we may have just helped create, not go off gallivanting from cave to cave looking for more "caveman cuddles" (to put it euphemistically). So prolactin and oxytocin (the bonding hormone you may have heard of) are released to encourage us to stick around. If you have never experienced SSRI-related sexual dysfunction, imagine that first five minutes post orgasm and you have an approximation of how it feels. However I should point out that this would be an extreme case and most patients either experience minimal impact or none at all.

Another problem with sertraline is, because of the way it is metabolised in your body, it can affect a range of different medications (either increasing or decreasing the effects of other drugs) like fluoxetine does. If you are taking medications for other conditions, you may need to discuss this with your doctor to ensure there is no interaction. In my experience, some doctors are not aware of all the interactions that sertraline has with other drugs, so you may need to be proactive and raise the topic yourself. I can't tell you the number of times I have heard from someone who has been started on an SSRI without the doctor realising that it may affect existing medications. As an example, sertraline can affect the metabolism of the blood-thinning drug warfarin. Considering what warfarin is used to treat, it is one of the last drugs I would ever want to inadvertently compromise. Another problem with this is that sertraline's effects on other drugs is the fact that, depending on the drug, sertraline can either increase or decrease its effects. So whereas sertraline inhibits the ability of warfarin to thin the blood, it can increase the effects of opiates and opioids such as methadone by almost 50%. Considering the dangers associated with opiate overdose, this risk is not insignificant. So if you are taking other medications, ask your doctor to check their drug database to see if there are any potential interactions you need to account for.

Citalopram & Escitalopram (*Cipramil, Lexapro*)

The reason why these two are listed together is that escitalopram is the updated version of citalopram, with the inactive part of citalopram removed to enable a lower dosage and therefore (in theory), a lower incidence of unwanted side-effects. Some researchers (including the developer of escitalopram), have also hypothesized that this inactive part of the compound actually inhibits the ability of the active component to boost serotonin. There are actually some interesting chemistry-related aspects to the difference between citalopram and escitalopram, with citalopram known as a racemic mixture and escitalopram being the left-enantiomer of citalopram. However I am conscious of the fact that the beginning of this book is already quite jargon-heavy, with some new concepts for some readers. So I won't cover the topic of isomers and racemic mixtures until later in the section on the SNRI milnacipran.

Escitalopram was developed in the late 90s and then largely superseded citalopram when it was approved by the FDA in 2002. However it would be remiss of me not to mention that there is some debate as to whether the newer variant is more effective or whether it is indeed associated with a lower incidence of side-effects. The philosophical and ethical debate is largely around the practice undertaken by pharmaceutical companies called *evergreening*, which is where they release a new drug which is only a slight variation of an existing drug. Then, as the older variant goes off-patent, they can release the updated version and therefore maintain the income stream.

I think that this is an important debate to have as a society as it can create an environment of perverse incentives. For example, the developers of citalopram may have known of its shortcomings and the fact that they could address this by releasing escitalopram from the get-go. They may have known that escitalopram would be more effective or have less side-effects, however by holding it back to focus on citalopram, they could in effect double the potential earning power of the drug – a difference of hundreds of millions or even billions of dollars. My personal opinion is that while I am sure that escitalopram was developed to extend the income-generating potential of citalopram, the general consensus among patients is that escitalopram *is* more effective.

However I understand that this is probably not a debate which someone reading this book should be focusing on at this point in time. So all I would recommend drawing from this is that escitalopram tends to equal citalopram's effectiveness at half the dose and is usually associated with a better side-effect profile. Whilst the usual dose targeted by doctors is 20mg, the right dose for you will be a function of your illness and its severity. For example, I know a lot of people who have found micro-dosing escitalopram (say, 2.5mg) to be an effective long-term maintenance dose which acts as a kind of preventative once they have recovered from major depression. This kind of dose could also be sufficient for mild-to-moderate cases of depression or GAD.

Like other SSRIs, I favour starting as low as possible and gradually titrating up to either 10mg or 20mg. If you see a remission of symptoms at 10mg, there is no hard and fast rule that you *must* keep going to 20mg. As mentioned earlier, OCD is the main exception, with much higher doses usually required. Earlier when I mentioned dosages as high as 80mg for fluoxetine, I did so as an example of the general ballpark difference between depression dosages and OCD dosages. As dosages of any SSRI start to increase beyond the mean, so too do complications such as side-effects. The treatment of OCD with drugs is therefore the sole domain of face-to-face interaction between you and your psychiatrist. So I will refrain from stating any "typical" dose of an SSRI for OCD beyond my earlier example. At these higher dosages, the dosage which works for you could be several orders of magnitude higher or lower than the typical dose.

So that leaves us with the most common question I hear regarding this particular SSRI – *Escitalopram or citalopram?*

In general, I tend to try escitalopram first, and if it doesn't work as expected, try one of the unrelated SSRIs such as sertraline. However, to counterbalance this, I should also point out that I have seen examples where citalopram worked better than escitalopram, despite the fact that there is no rational explanation for why this would be the case. Have I mentioned that brains are weird yet?

For a while after escitalopram was released and citalopram went off-patent, there was a compelling financial reason to stick with citalopram as it became a much cheaper option. However both escitalopram and citalopram are now off-patent so there should be no cost difference any more.

From this point on I will refer to escitalopram due to both the pharmacological equivalence and the fact that citalopram is rarely used now. However most of the following holds true for both.

Escitalopram is the most selective of all the SSRIs, having potent serotonergic effects and insignificant effects on other neurotransmitters, thus a virtual absence of activity at dopaminergic, adrenergic, histamine and cholinergic receptors. In other words, if your problem is purely serotonin related, escitalopram will give you the most "laser-targeted" results.

Based on this level of selectivity and relative freedom from adverse side-effects, escitalopram has slowly become the "gold standard" SSRI favoured by doctors as a safe, effective first option. It must be noted however, that escitalopram is still associated with the same side-effects as other SSRIs, such as sexual dysfunction and sleep disturbances. Of these, escitalopram tends to cause sexual side-effects slightly more often than other SSRIs, which is likely a function of its selectivity for serotonin.

The price to pay for such selective amplification of serotonin is usually suppressed dopamine activity, and suppressed dopamine activity usually equals suppressed libido.

Fluvoxamine (*Luvox*)

Fluvoxamine is another potential SSRI to consider, however it is generally believed to have no particular advantage over other SSRIs apart from its approval to be used to treat OCD. Thus, unless you have OCD, your doctor would usually favour alternatives before considering fluvoxamine. That's not to say that it isn't effective, just that it has no particular "killer feature" justifying its use as a first-line treatment for mood disorders.

That said, it is worth noting that often this is more a question of marketing than anything else. All SSRIs are proven to be effective for OCD (and conversely, fluvoxamine is effective as an antidepressant), so the developers of fluvoxamine have apparently decided that their marketing angle to compete with other SSRIs is to pitch it as an OCD medication.

Despite this, clomipramine remains the gold standard in the treatment of OCD. What this means is that clomipramine should be more effective, but with significantly worse side-effects for some. So if you have OCD and clomipramine isn't an option, fluvoxamine may be a useful backup. Or, another way of looking at it is that fluvoxamine would be a worthy first-line treatment for mild-to-moderate OCD because the side-effects of clomipramine might not be worth it. However for severe, disabling OCD, clomipramine remains favoured by most doctors.

Aside from its action on serotonin, the main distinguishing feature of fluvoxamine is that, like sertraline, it also functions as sigma (σ_1) receptor agonist. The sigma receptor largely remains a mystery, however many researchers believe that it is involved in mood disorders in some way, and activating this receptor tends to reduce anxiety and improve mood. All I can say about sigma receptor agonists is that they work, but we have no idea why. However expect this to change over the next few years as research advances. Within the next few years I fully expect to be able to update my position on sigma receptor agonism.

Another one of my "*things doctors don't tell you but should*" points on fluvoxamine is that its metabolism is significantly altered in patients who smoke. If you are a smoker, you may need a dose which is at least 20% more than a non-smoker. While on the subject of metabolism, it is again important to note that, like other SSRIs, it affects the liver enzymes which metabolise other drugs. Fluvoxamine affects almost all of the major sub-types of these enzymes, creating a high probability that it will affect other drugs you are taking. The list of drugs affected by fluvoxamine is huge, and depending on the drug, fluvoxamine can either increase or decrease its potency so please discussion with your doctor.

The metabolism of fluvoxamine is also important in terms of its half-life, which, due to being slightly less than 24 hours, means that many doctors prefer twice-daily dosing to ensure that levels remain stable.

Paroxetine *(Paxil)*

Paroxetine is the single most potent SSRI in terms of effects on serotonin, so naturally you would expect it to be the "go-to" option for moderate to severe cases. You may therefore be surprised to learn that these days it is prescribed less and less, with doctors preferring escitalopram and sertraline as first-line options for a few reasons.

Firstly, paroxetine is associated with particularly unpleasant discontinuation syndrome which makes it a difficult drug to withdraw from for many people. In particular, paroxetine is known for causing "electric-shock" like symptoms known as *brain-zaps* when people reduce their dose too quickly. According to many anecdotal reports, this can be an incredibly unpleasant experience. In addition, withdrawing from paroxetine can also feature some of the more typical SSRI withdrawal symptoms such as nausea, insomnia, dizziness and a temporary spike in anxiety or depressed mood. These symptoms tend to be more intense with paroxetine withdrawal than other SSRIs.

It is thought that another reason why paroxetine can be problematic to withdraw from is because of a pharmacokinetic quirk specific to itself only, among SSRIs. Paroxetine appears to inhibit its own metabolism when dosed chronically. By inhibiting this process, it becomes more difficult for your body to clear it out of your system, perhaps contributing to its potency. However when you start withdrawing, a kind of snowball effect is created where there is no longer sufficient levels in your system to inhibit clearance, speeding up the process as a result. The only way to mitigate this is to taper down very slowly and very carefully.

A surprising number of doctors are unaware that there is a controlled-release form of paroxetine (often marketed as *Paxil CR*) which may be a better initial option, as well as providing a useful tool for withdrawing. Prior to beginning your taper off the drug, a good strategy may be to switch to the controlled-release form which may make the process easier to manage.

However another reason why many doctors eschew paroxetine is due to its unfortunate notoriety, which is a result of its developer (GlaxoSmithKline – GSK) being fined USD$3 billion dollars by the US Department of Justice for misrepresenting its efficacy. According to the Department of Justice –

> *"The United States alleges that, among other things, GSK participated in preparing, publishing and distributing a misleading medical journal article that misreported that a clinical trial of Paxil demonstrated efficacy in the treatment of depression in patients under age 18, when the study failed to demonstrate efficacy."*

This is just the kind of unethical practice which "Big Pharma" is notorious for, weakening the general public's already sceptical view of antidepressants and playing into the hands of those claiming that drugs are ineffective or dangerous.

However if it turns out that paroxetine is the best drug for you, take solace in the knowledge that it has already gone off-patent, so none of your money will find its way to GSK.

Now that we have the negatives out of the way, let's have a look at some of the more positive aspects of paroxetine.

Paroxetine's withdrawal symptoms would be a deal-breaker if it was an ineffective drug, however that is far from the case, with this drawback being just one side of what is a double-edged sword. One of the reasons why it is so difficult to withdraw from paroxetine is due to its serotonergic potency. And it is for this reason that paroxetine can be particularly helpful in cases of severe anxiety or OCD. For some people, when all else fails, paroxetine proves to be the one medication that provides relief from their symptoms. Therefore, despite its shortcomings, paroxetine should not be completely discarded as an option. It is worth remembering that in severe cases, some form of medication (be it paroxetine or otherwise) will be required indefinitely. In cases such as these, paroxetine's withdrawal symptoms become largely irrelevant, as there will be no need to stop.

Naturally, the flip-side of this is that paroxetine would most likely be inappropriate for moderate or time-limited cases, as a protracted and unpleasant withdrawal process could imperil the progress made up until that point.

In terms of pharmacology, apart from its potent serotonergic effects, paroxetine is notable for possessing mild noradrenaline reuptake inhibition, although nowhere near the degree seen with SNRIs (which I will cover next). Paroxetine is also the only SSRI which possesses anticholinergic activity,

Of all the SSRI's, paroxetine tends to be the most anxiety-specific drug, rarely being used specifically for major depression. Naturally this lends itself to use in OCD treatment, which usually requires the kind of serotonergic potency which paroxetine wields. However it can be an effective treatment across the spectrum of anxiety disorders. For example, an expert I work with believes that paroxetine is the single most effective SSRI for the treatment of social anxiety.

Finally, I should mention that paroxetine also affects the metabolism of other drugs in a similar fashion to most other SSRIs, so discuss any potential interactions with your doctor.

As you would no doubt have gleaned from their name, SNRIs are essentially SSRIs with an additional mode of action, which is to also inhibit the reuptake of noradrenaline, leading to higher levels remaining in the synapse.

Over the course of the 20th century there were distinct periods where a single neurotransmitter would become the main focus of psychopharmacology. Invariably, researchers would then turn their attention elsewhere, only to then return to the neurotransmitter in question, several decades later. When you compress this process down to a paragraph of exposition, researchers start to sound like herd animals with ADHD. Many people don't realise that, in the era before SSRIs, for a long time noradrenaline was believed to be the central player in depression. Most people are shocked to hear that, in the dawn of this nascent discipline, amphetamines were a common first-line treatment for depressive disorders.

However, with the advent of the SSRI, which began with the development of fluoxetine (Prozac), noradrenaline was consigned to the scrap heap and all focus shifted to serotonin. Fortunately, we now appear to have entered into an era where the complex interplay of various neurotransmitters is properly acknowledged. However this is at the research level. To this day, the vast majority of patients with mood disorders will leave their doctor's office with a script for an SSRI, so clearly we have not reached the stage where new discoveries are influencing prescribing habits.

In the pre-SSRI, for a long time, tricyclic antidepressants (TCAs) were the standard first-line treatment for anxiety and depression. As I will explain later when I cover this class of drugs, TCAs are essentially SNRIs, but with a long list of secondary actions. Some of these actions contribute to their effectiveness, while others are unwanted and end up being a trigger for the patient discontinuing treatment. Other effects, such as their impact on cardiovascular health, can create risks for the patient. In a pre-SSRI world, these risks were seen as an acceptable trade-off, with most patients happy to put up with weight gain or a dry mouth and doctors comfortable with the cardiovascular risk, if the net effect was the alleviation of mental suffering. However, with the appearance of SSRIs on the scene, with their much "cleaner" pharmacological profile, TCAs were viewed as anachronistic.

So it should come as no surprise to learn that once drug companies each had their own "blockbuster" SSRI, attention then turned to developing variants which also boosted noradrenaline, yet were not associated with the drawbacks of TCAs. Soon after (well, at least in the context of drug development, which can be a long process) we saw venlafaxine (Effexor) as the first product of this research. This was then followed by several more SNRIs with slightly different pharmacological profiles.

---

[7] Serotonin-*noradrenaline* reuptake inhibitor in certain countries.

The question - *SSRI or SNRI?* – is a common one which, as you probably guessed, comes down to the individual. As a class, SNRIs enjoy a modest advantage over SSRIs when meta-analyses are conducted. However, as there is such huge variation between the individual drugs in each class, along with a patient's response to these drugs, this comparison becomes rather meaningless.

In the vast majority of cases, doctors will make a fairly simplistic assessment of whether someone is anxious, anxiously depressed or lethargically depressed, before deciding on whether an SSRI or an SNRI would be appropriate. This means that, in general, an SNRI will figure in your doctor's thinking if you report a lack of energy as part of your depression.

In effect, this means that many people with anxiety disorders are steered away from SNRIs because of their noradrenaline-boosting effects, as extra noradrenaline can sometimes exacerbate anxiety. However in reality, things are a little less straightforward as noradrenaline, like serotonin and dopamine, is a complex neurotransmitter. In reality, noradrenaline defies any simplistic causal association with anxiety or panic. To expand on my earlier explanation, if you are overjoyed about something (say, your partner just proposed marriage, or you just won the lottery, for example) and you then were given a drug which instantaneously boosted levels of noradrenaline, it would most likely just make you more viscerally excited, accentuating your good mood. However, if you had just had the opposite occur (say, you were just told you have only months to live, or something equally awful), this hypothetical noradrenaline drug could trigger intense anxiety or even panic.

If you were to talk to a neuroscientist, they would no doubt say that even this example oversimplifies things. They would want to know *which areas* of your brain were affected by this hypothetical drug before they would be comfortable predicting the emotional effects. Depending on the areas involved, this spike in noradrenaline could help a child with ADHD focus or it could cause a panic attack.

This is actually an incredibly important point more broadly. Simply having high or low levels of noradrenaline tells us very little about your mood or anxiety levels. We need to know where (in the brain) and when (the context) to predict the effects of noradrenaline. In this sense, it is almost like turning the volume knob up on your emotions. If you were unable to produce noradrenaline, winning the lottery wouldn't feel as great and hearing about your impending demise would pack less emotional punch. Often with anxiety and depression, this context-sensing apparatus becomes faulty, often leading to any increase in noradrenaline being interpreted as unpleasant.

I addressed this point in detail in my book The Excitement Principle, where I detailed how I overcame my fear of public speaking. Before an important speaking engagement, someone without an anxiety disorder may find the high arousal state "exciting" or "thrilling", however someone with an anxiety disorder (and more

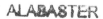

specifically, a public speaking phobia) would find the exact same physical symptoms extremely unpleasant. One of the things I recommend people address (either on their own or with an expert in CBT) is to work on gradually becoming comfortable with this high adrenaline state. This process can require patience, as you are sometimes attempting to unlearn years (if not decades) of mental associations.

This ability of noradrenaline to add flavour to, or enhance the intensity of our experiences is best exemplified by recent research into post-traumatic stress disorder (PTSD). Researchers have found that if you give someone a beta-blocker such as propranolol immediately following a traumatic experience, it can often short-circuit the process whereby this experience morphs into PTSD. Beta-blockers block the ability of noradrenaline and adrenaline to activate *beta-adrenergic* receptors which mediate your fight or flight response. Researchers believe that, in this context, noradrenaline is used to establish the emotional weight of certain memories. By blocking this process after a traumatic event, instead of the memory being encoded as *"this is the most important/devastating/traumatic thing that has ever happened to me"*, is it stored in your hippocampus with the neural equivalent of *"meh"*.

So, to return to SNRIs specifically, sometimes they can be helpful because their serotonergic effects help reframe your perception in a more positive light and the noradrenergic effects can help recharge your batteries which have been drained by a long period of anxiety and stress. One of the things people are often surprised to hear is the fact that noradrenaline has a major role to play in how you handle stress. People assume that, because they are stressed, they need to suppress noradrenaline. However in addressing this topic it is important to distinguish acute effects and chronic effects, as well as the need to distinguish between *nor*adrenaline and adrenaline. Rather than getting lost in pages of unnecessary minutiae, let's just distil this topic down to –

- Noradrenaline's job is to keep you alive when something happens which your brain perceives as potentially dangerous.
- Noradrenaline does a wonderful job when the stress is acute (you are being chased by a dangerous animal), but less so when the stress is chronic (each month you wonder how you are going to pay the bills, you are in an abusive relationship)
- In day to day situation, your brain uses noradrenaline to direct behaviour by attaching an emotional flavour to certain activities. If something bad happens, noradrenaline makes it "feel" bad so we avoid it in future. If something good happens, noradrenaline makes it "feel" great, thereby guiding us towards repeating it.

So, to then apply this to SNRIs, a simplified way of looking at this is that they can help restore normal noradrenaline levels which may have been depleted after a period of chronic stress. Whilst the start-up period can often be associated with worse transient anxiety than SSRIs, once you begin experiencing therapeutic effects, they can often *reduce* anxiety. By restoring normal activity, you should then start seeing better stress tolerance, increased focus (inability to concentrate is one of the most common symptoms of depression and anxiety disorders) and the return of "colour" to your day.

This last point is crucial. Most people who have never experienced depression first-hand assume that it involves intense emotional states such as profound sadness or fear. Whilst these states can form a central part of an individual's depression, in moderate-to-severe cases, the problem is not intense emotions but the complete absence of *any* emotion, good or bad. Many people report feeling "dead" inside, like all the colour and flavour have been sucked out of their world. I have found that these are the cases where an SNRI may have the edge over an SSRI. The extra noradrenaline can help "jump-start" people out of this colourless funk, restoring the normal highs and lows of our human existence.

As mentioned previously, this process of matching symptoms to surpluses or deficits of certain neurotransmitters is far from an exact science – particularly where there are mixed anxiety/emotional flatness states. However it can, at the very least, give you some clarity around your symptoms so that you are able to provide insightful commentary to your doctor when deciding on treatment options.

Another important factor which could contribute to the decision-making process is whether pain is a factor. This is one area where SNRIs have a clear advantage over SSRIs, as they can also act as effective painkillers. For example, duloxetine is one of the only medications that is FDA-approved for treating fibromyalgia. I have found that there is an enormous crossover between mood disorders and various manifestations of pain. Depending on the type of pain, this can be the typical aches and pains seen in major depression, such as stomach aches and headaches, or disorders such as fibromyalgia which have considerable overlap with mood disorders.

The reason why SNRIs treat pain is complex. To use the same analogy from a moment ago, if you imagine your brain having a tank for each neurotransmitter, chronic stress can literally drain your neurotransmitter reserves. Neurotransmitters like serotonin and noradrenaline play an important role in modulating your perception of pain.

It is no coincidence that most people suffering from anxiety or depression first visit their doctor due to physical pain, rather than the psychological component. This is an important point to note. You may be surprised to hear that, in my experience, many people notice the physical pain before the psychological pain. An experienced doctor will always have this in the back of their mind if you complain of vague aches and pains. And in particular, aches and pains which don't respond to OTC pain-relievers such as ibuprofen. If you have a physical injury of some kind, the pain is largely caused by inflammation around the site of the injury. So if an anti-inflammatory doesn't do anything, it should at the very least cause the doctor to inquire as to your current mental state or whether you have been under unusually high levels of stress.

Unfortunately there is still a lot we don't know regarding the role which different neurotransmitters play in *nociception* (the feeling of pain). We know that serotonin plays at least some role, however SSRIs typically don't perform well as pain-relievers, whereas SNRIs do. So this then brings the role of noradrenaline into focus. Again, by taking an evolutionary viewpoint, this becomes quite logical. If we return to our discussion around the role inflammation plays in stress (your brain thinks stress=danger=potential injury), it makes sense that the main neurotransmitter which helps you fight or flee would also help dull any pain which may result.

The other reason why mood disorders (and in particular, anxiety disorders) are associated with pain is that an anxious person will go through their day unconsciously clenching their muscles tight. Some anxious people I meet have shoulders which feel like rock! This constant tension can then start to manifest as back pain or tension headaches.

Now let's move on to the specific SNRIs. One point I would like to first make is that each SNRI is markedly different from the others. When it boils down to it, each SSRI works roughly the same as the other SSRIs, with only incremental differences. However the SNRIs are each quite distinctive, making the choice easier once the diagnosis is known.

Venlafaxine/Desvenlafaxine (*Effexor/Pristiq*)

Venlafaxine is a powerful and widely used SNRI which is often prescribed for severe depression, particularly where there is a lethargic component which may benefit from the added noradrenaline reuptake inhibition. When all else fails, many doctors turn to venlafaxine due to its dual properties and potent action. In recent years, venlafaxine has waned in popularity at the expense of duloxetine. This is due to the fact that duloxetine also has the added benefit of treating neuropathic pain, so while duloxetine is more widely prescribed, a large proportion of this is its use as a treatment for fibromyalgia. This makes for a relatively simple decision if your doctor favours an SNRI. If there is a pain component they will usually go for duloxetine and for "pure" lethargic depression, venlafaxine is often favoured.

Like escitalopram is to citalopram, *des*venlafaxine is the 'updated' version of venlafaxine. There is debate as to how much of an improvement the newer version is over the older version, however it is difficult to gauge as the uptake of desvenlafaxine has not been strong by doctors and their patients, making statistical comparisons unwise. Unfortunately I have found that the general view among clinicians is that desvenlafaxine has been rather disappointing in terms of its effectiveness versus the older version. From a purely biological or neurochemical perspective I find this surprising, as desvenlafaxine is just the "active" metabolite of venlafaxine, so you would expect the effects to be similar, however for whatever reason, it appears as if this is not the case.

However there is an assumption here which may provide at least some explanation. I have assumed that desvenlafaxine is *the* only active metabolite of venlafaxine. Perhaps there are other metabolites of venlafaxine which contribute to its clinical effects or to the side-effect profile.

In fact, theoretically desvenlafaxine overcomes one of the shortcomings of its older sibling. One of the peculiarities of venlafaxine is that at lower doses, it works mostly as an SSRI (that is, with minimal impact on noradrenaline), due largely to the fact that venlafaxine's serotonergic effects are five-times more potent than its effects on noradrenaline. Then, once a certain dosage threshold is reached, venlafaxine begins affecting noradrenaline as well. In-vitro studies have indicated that desvenlafaxine overcomes this issue, boosting noradrenaline even at low doses, so its modest reputation in the real-world has always surprised me. Again, however, at the risk of sounding like a broken record, it is important to note the distinction between a drug's general reputation and its benefit (or lack thereof) for you. In this sense, against every possible metric except for "average user feedback", the newer version stacks up favourably.

The general consensus is that 75mg of venlafaxine would be a sensible starting point to taper up from. As I tend to favour starting at half the usual starting point, don't be afraid to cut or break your pills in half to start at 37.5mg. An exception here is the controlled release form (which I cover in a moment) as controlled release tablets should never be broken because their time-release mechanism usually involves the outer layer of the tablet acting as an enteric coating[8]. The other consensus is that true SNRI effects don't manifest until 150mg or so. While most patients respond to 10-20mg of escitalopram, the dosage ranges seen with venlafaxine can be much wider, so for more serious cases, your doctor may target 300mg and beyond.

Venlafaxine's lack of SNRI properties at low doses means that it is not really an ideal option for more "moderate" cases which may only require modest dosages. In most cases, using venlafaxine at dosages below 150mg defeats the purpose of choosing an SNRI over an SSRI.

However there is definitely one group of people who will respond better to the newer version. As mentioned earlier, antidepressants are almost all metabolised by certain liver enzymes. One of these enzymes is the unimaginatively named CYP2D6, whose main claim to fame (apart from being confused with droid who associates with Luke Skywalker) is the fact that it is perhaps *the* major player in SSRI/SNRI metabolism. However there is a sub-group of the general population who genetically lack this enzyme (or, at the very least, have impaired function). As this is the main enzyme needed to clear venlafaxine from the body, people with impaired CYP2D6 function will often experience a much higher incidence of side-effects. If you are one of these people, desvenlafaxine should be the better option in terms of side-effect profile.

Before I move on, this is an opportune time to mention the fact that you can have a test conducted to elucidate whether you have impaired function for any of the major liver enzymes. Whilst purely optional, if you have the financial resources or healthcare coverage, it can, at the very least, be a way of eliminating certain drugs from contention. I have included more information on this topic in the Appendix.

One final distinction between how these two drugs are metabolised is that venlafaxine's metabolism can be affected by drugs which inhibit the *P-glycoprotein transporter*, whereas desvenlafaxine isn't. This transporter molecule has a similar function to cytochrome P450 enzymes, constantly working to hunt down what it believes are "toxins", escorting them "out of the building" via what I will euphemistically called "excretory mechanisms". Drugs which inhibit this process can then change how much of other drugs you absorb. This is one of the reasons why you cannot take the herbal antidepressant St. John's Wort with other drugs, as it inhibits this clearing process.

What this means in effect is that desvenlafaxine would be preferable for patients taking other drugs at the same time. While the chances of you taking a pure P-glycoprotein inhibitor at the same time as you begin antidepressant therapy are slim,

---

[8] Some time-release tablets employ a matrix-style system to slow absorption, meaning they retain their time-release function even when broken.

a huge number of drugs have at least some effects on either this transporter molecule or P450 enzymes. Some inhibit these enzymes, while other induce them, creating an added layer of unpredictability which is unhelpful when trying to establish an effective drug therapy and dosage.

The main downside of venlafaxine is its notoriously difficult discontinuation profile. Venlafaxine is widely reputed to be one of the hardest antidepressants to stop, due to both its dual-action and its relatively short half-life. A potentially useless piece of trivia is that venlafaxine is almost identical to the painkiller tramadol (which I will cover later in the book) in terms of its chemical structure, with tramadol's mild opiate activity being the main difference. However, interestingly, there is some evidence that venlafaxine possesses some indirect opioid activity which might contribute to both its usefulness in mood disorders and pain states. One interesting aspect of this similarity is that both venlafaxine and tramadol are widely reported to be two of the most difficult drugs to stop taking, due to their sometimes brutal discontinuation symptoms. The other interesting aspect of this is that tramadol is sometimes used as an antidepressant of last resort, when other options have failed.

Due to its relatively short half-life, venlafaxine should be avoided in cases where there is a likelihood that doses will be forgotten (e.g. – where there is significant cognitive impairment, or in geriatric settings) or where it will be inconvenient to re-dose more than once a day, due to work commitments or in a school setting, for example). However I should also mention that there is an extended release version of venlafaxine (sold as Effexor XR in many markets) available which enables once-daily dosing.

Surprisingly, despite the obvious appeal from a convenience standpoint, I have found that many prefer the instant release form for whatever reason. If a decision is made to start venlafaxine, I often recommend people to try the extended release form or desvenlafaxine as the first option. I have heard first-hand reports from patients taking venlafaxine who complain that if they miss their dose for whatever reason, a highly unpleasant withdrawal can start as little as two hours later. Considering the multitude of factors which can precipitate a missed dose, this strikes me as an unnecessary risk considering the availability of extended release forms and countless other antidepressants.

For me, this highlights a broader issue. Where possible, I always recommend to people that once they are stable on a drug which works well, the drug needs to fade into the background to allow you to get on with life. Naturally, the means that it would be inadvisable for you to ruminate on the topic of antidepressants all day. People can sometimes become overly obsessive about this topic, constantly returning to their doctor to change drugs because of something they read or heard. Or spending their days on online depression-related forums. The danger with this is that you can gradually start defining yourself subconsciously as "as a depressed person taking medication". This is because we are talking about the brain, not some other body part. If you lost an arm, you would still be "you". However the same cannot be said for your brain, for obvious reasons. Just like when you need to take antibiotics for an infection, you are not defined by the antibiotics, your antidepressant should be "just something you take" and should not be allowed to figure prominently in your daily thoughts.

It is for this reason that I am not typically a fan of antidepressants which require multiple doses throughout the day. Not only does it make it harder to keep your medication from infiltrating your day, I can't help but feel these drugs enslave you somewhat. You can end up avoiding certain activities where you know you may be unable to re-dose discreetly.

Back to venlafaxine, the other advantage of the controlled-release form is that it will be significantly easier to withdraw from down the track if and when a decision is made to discontinue. Alternatively, if you take the instant release form and wish to stop, you could consider first switching to the controlled-release form before tapering. Irrespective of which form you take, extreme caution should be taken to withdraw slowly, reducing the dose by small amounts each week. Alternatively, you may discuss with your doctor the option of switching to fluoxetine first, before tapering, to reduce the discomfort associated with venlafaxine withdrawal. As mentioned earlier, fluoxetine's long half-life gives it an in-built taper as the drug leaves your system very slowly.

For more information on stopping your antidepressant, check out my guide in the appendix.

One of the most interesting uses for venlafaxine is as a combination therapy with mirtazapine (which I will cover in the next section) interestingly called *California Rocket Fuel*. The combination of an SNRI with a receptor agonist/antagonist appears to, in the words of Bing Crosby, *"accentuate the positives and eliminate the negatives"* of venlafaxine as a monotherapy. The combination of these two drugs can lead to double the remission rate[9] usually seen when either of these drugs are used alone.

---

[9]*Remission in this context meaning the depression is successfully treated either permanently or at least temporarily)*

Duloxetine *(Cymbalta)*

While duloxetine is also used for depression and anxiety, it tends to find most of its use as an effective treatment for fibromyalgia and other forms of neuropathic pain. If you have depression or anxiety along with neuropathic pain, duloxetine should be one of the first options for consideration. In terms of efficacy, duloxetine is roughly similar to venlafaxine, but without the strange dose-dependent effects on noradrenaline. Duloxetine has a linear dose-response regarding effects on serotonin and noradrenaline, which means it is probably the closest drug we have to a "prototypical" SNRI.

Another difference between these two SNRIs is that duloxetine tends to have worse side-effects at the beginning of treatment, however once the drug has begun to take effect after 4-6 weeks, both duloxetine and venlafaxine have similar side effects when they are both taken at the recommended dosages.

In practical terms, the main difference between duloxetine and venlafaxine is that duloxetine is still covered by patent (with some exceptions, mentioned in a moment), which unfortunately means that it is quite expensive compared to other options and is not available in many different dosages. It is only available in a standard 60mg dose or a "starting" 30mg dose[10], in capsule form. I have never been a fan of drugs in capsules as it makes it impossible to cut into smaller doses with a pill cutter. This makes slow titration up (when starting) or slow taper down (when finishing) more difficult. Hopefully when this drug goes off-patent there will be a wider range of options. I can't help but think that the lack of dose options and scored tablets is financially motivated in some way. I see an identical issue with one of Pfizer's patent-protected drugs, pregabalin (Lyrica). For example, for both pregabalin and duloxetine, both dosages cost roughly equal, so if they were supplied as scored tablets, patients could split a higher dose in two, effectively halving the cost. However this becomes incredibly time consuming and fiddly if you wanted to do the same thing with capsules.

The good news is that duloxetine has started going off-patent in certain markets, which should open up the dosage options. However you will need to check its status in your country. For example, some generic forms have recently become available in the USA but not in Australia. In certain markets, the reason for the delay is that the developers of duloxetine, Eli Lilly, obtained a 6 month extension of their patent protection. To give you an idea of the amounts of money involved in a decision like this (and therefore the perfect environment for lobbyists to be able to influence government policy), this 6 month extension of duloxetine's protection alone was worth $1.5 billion for the company.

---

[10] The 30mg dose is made available by Pfizer to enable titration up and down when starting or finishing duloxetine.

While the withdrawal from duloxetine is not as famously difficult as venlafaxine, you can still expect it to be at least as difficult as SSRI withdrawal and possibly worse, because noradrenaline is also involved.

In terms of safety, duloxetine is broadly similar to other SSRIs and SNRIs except for one important exception. When duloxetine is metabolised (by CYP1A2 and CYP2D6) in the liver, it produces a metabolite which can be toxic for some people. It is therefore contraindicated for alcoholics, former alcoholics and those with liver diseases such as cirrhosis or fatty liver. I can find no evidence that duloxetine presents any danger for patients not meeting this criteria. Also, just briefly, while we are on the subject of its metabolism, I should point out that if you are taking other drugs which affect CYP1A2 and CYP2D6, it may affect your response to duloxetine. And similar to other SSRIs and SNRIs, duloxetine is itself a potent inhibitor of CYP1A2.

In terms of potency, at the standard 60mg dosage, duloxetine would be towards the higher end of the spectrum. For example, its effects on serotonin reuptake are significantly more potent than fluoxetine (which is the mildest of the SSRIs) and it also has its effects on noradrenaline on top of this. Despite this, the performance of duloxetine in clinical trials for depression is surprisingly unimpressive. For example, a Cochrane review[11] in 2012 found that duloxetine performed no better than existing SSRIs, despite the added noradrenaline boost. In fact, in their review, this difference in pharmacology was likely to be a key driver in their assessment that duloxetine is associated with slightly worse side-effects than the SSRIs it was being compared against. Of these, nausea, headache and dry mouth tend to feature prominently. Considering this, I don't typically view duloxetine as one of the first drugs I would be looking at for the treatment of depression or anxiety disorders.

In addition to the side-effects reported in clinical trials, I can add one more bit of real-world input. In those I have worked with and across the various online discussion groups I researched as part of this book, one side-effect seems to be mentioned more than any other – sweating. The tendency of duloxetine to make some people sweat profusely is one of the most common reasons given for why they quit taking it. Perhaps the group of people who should most heed this warning is menopausal women who are suffering from hot flashes, as, in my experience the combination of hot flashes and profuse sweating is far from enjoyable. On my own person list of "Things I don't enjoy", this combination features somewhere near the bottom, alongside "anything involving Justin Bieber".

However where duloxetine's appeal increases is where there is also a neuropathic pain component, such as diabetic peripheral neuropathy or fibromyalgia. In particular, due to a significant crossover and co-morbidity, it is cases where there is

---

[11] Cochrane is an independent network of researchers and health professionals which conducts the most trusted meta-analyses, where they pool all the available data on certain drugs.

fibromyalgia plus depression or anxiety where duloxetine has solid evidence. To be even more specific, cases such as the above where no other medications are currently being taken or cases where there is patient resistance to poly-drug therapies (where the patient has no desire to be on multiple drugs at the same time). In highly technical terms, this strategy is known in psychopharmacology as *two birds with one stone.*

However, here's the thing. Purely as an antidepressant or anxiolytic, duloxetine is just run of the mill, and purely as a pain-reliever it is also run of the mill. I put the proportion of people who receive pain relief at 50% (at best). And of these, most only achieve modest reductions in pain levels. In my experience, for mixed depression/anxiety/fibromyalgia, an SSRI plus drugs such as tramadol[12], pregabalin or memantine tends to meet with more success.

However, apart from their tendency to occur together, the other thing fibromyalgia has in common with anxiety or depression is that they are all caused by a huge number of different factors which vary wildly from person to person. I have read clinical trials on duloxetine for fibromyalgia which were positively glowing, as well as countless user experiences to the same effect. And I have also read lukewarm data and seen many patients complain that they experienced no benefits whatsoever. This appears to be the very situation for which the acronym *YMMV (your mileage may vary)* was created.

What concerns me most about the use of duloxetine in fibromyalgia is the potential for drug/drug interactions, due to its clearance from the body being affected by liver enzymes and the fact that it is itself a strong inhibitor of CYP1A2. The average fibromyalgia patient currently takes between 3-6 different drugs per day. There is a high likelihood that most, if not all, of these drugs are metabolised via the cytochrome P450 system, so the introduction of duloxetine has the potential to cause problematic changes to how these drugs are absorbed and cleared from the body.

One final point, which may or may not be relevant in your case, is that I saw a study which found that duloxetine increased levels of dopamine in the pre-frontal cortex. As duloxetine has no direct effects on dopamine, in all likelihood it achieves this by boosting noradrenaline (increasing one tends to pull the other one up too, as opposed to serotonin, which tends to be suppressed by the other two), something which the other SNRIs would also achieve in all probability. More interesting is the *where* component of this story, as increased dopamine in the pre-frontal cortex tends to have little direct impact on mood. For dopamine to give you pleasure and

---

[12] A word of caution. On Wikipedia and various discussion forums, potentially the most overstated risk would be serotonin syndrome. So many people are cautioned against taking an SSRI with tramadol. While there is never any such thing as a risk-free combination, experts I have spoken to have indicated that this is a combination used commonly with no issues. At the end of the day, whether this is a possible combination for you will depend on what your specialist is comfortable with, so please discuss it with them.

excitement, it needs to be boosted in the "pleasure centres" of the brain, such as the nucleus accumbens. However boosting dopamine in the pre-frontal cortex is one of the core targets of therapies used to treat attentional disorders such as ADHD and ADD, as it can boost cognitive processing, planning and memory retention.

Why am I telling you this? Well, like fibromyalgia, there is significant co-morbidity between ADHD/ADD and mood disorders such as anxiety and depression. So, if we were to return to our *two birds with one stone* analogy, while duloxetine might not be the best option if depression or anxiety is your only issue, if you have both a mood disorder *and* an attentional disorder, duloxetine may be worth further investigation.

Milnacipran & Levomilnacipran *(Savella/Ixel/Fetzima)*

Milnacipran is an SNRI primarily used in the treatment of fibromyalgia, where it provides comparable pain relief to duloxetine. Despite the fact that, on the surface there is little to distinguish milnacipran from its more widely-used SNRI brethren, in many countries (such as the USA) it is not approved as a treatment for depression. However you shouldn't interpret this as milnacipran not being effective for depression, or even anxiety. It just depends on your own individual mix of neurotransmitters and metabolism.

Whilst milnacipran is clearly a "me too" drug with what appears to be questionable differences to existing SNRIs, if you dig slightly below the surface, it does have some relatively unique properties. Of these, most important is the fact that it boosts noradrenaline much more potently than serotonin. Whereas duloxetine is fairly balanced and venlafaxine only starts affecting noradrenaline at higher doses, milnacipran has noradrenaline reuptake three times the strength of its serotonin reuptake.

What makes this particularly interesting is that until the development of milnacipran, if you required this particular mix of effects, your only option would be one of the noradrenaline-centric tricyclics (TCA), such as desipramine or nortriptyline. And in the handful of trials where milnacipran was compared to a TCA, the effectiveness was similar, however with the TCA there were significantly more dropouts (people quitting the trial due to intolerable side-effects). This means that the "ideal" patient for milnacipran is someone with a combination of major depression and fibromyalgia, who had previously responded well to a TCA but had to quit due to side-effects.

Another factor which distinguishes milnacipran is the way it is absorbed and cleared from your body. As mentioned earlier, most antidepressants rely on the cytochrome P450 system in the liver for being metabolised. However milnacipran is processed by the kidneys (to then be excreted in your urine) and by another hepatic (liver controlled) process known as *glucuronidation*. In effect, this means that milnacipran is free of the various pharmacokinetic complexities and risks seen with other antidepressants, making the combination of milnacipran with other medications less complicated.

As you may recall from the earlier section on escitalopram, I mentioned that I would revisit this concept later in the book. The development of the drug levomilnacipran gives us the perfect excuse to briefly cover this topic. If your eyes glaze over at the first hint of chemistry-talk, you may wish to skip several chapters ahead.

In chemistry, certain molecules are known as *stereoisomers*, which means they are made up of two halves called enantiomers which are effectively mirror images of each other. Like your face in a mirror, each enantiomer is made of the same basic material, but flipped. If a drug is one of these enantiomers, it is *dextrorotary* if it is the right-hand side enantiomer and *levorotary* if it is the left-hand side enantiomer. If the drug features both sides, it is known as a *racemic* mixture. These drugs are usually easy to spot because of their *dextro* or *levo* prefixes. The classic example is amphetamine, which is a racemic mixture made up of dextroamphetamine and levoamphetamine. The most widely used amphetamine in the USA is the drug brand Adderall, which, by using amphetamine salts creates a unique mixture which is 75% dextroamphetamine and 25% levoamphetamine. As the levo form tends to be less euphoric and more slanted towards noradrenaline related focus, this combination is particularly effective for treating ADHD[13]. More on amphetamine in the "off-label" treatment options.

However more specifically looking at antidepressants, citalopram/escitalopram was the first SSRI (if we view them as a single drug) which was released with one eye firmly on the potential for a drug company to use stereoisomers as a way of doubling the length of time a particular drug could continue generating profits for the developer. Citalopram was first released as a racemic mixture, so the idea that the drug's developer had no idea that the left enantiomer (escitalopram) might be more effective from the beginning seems a little improbable.

Keeping this in mind, if I were to tell you that milnacipran is a racemic mixture, I will give you one guess as to what its developers "suddenly" discovered after it had been on the market for a few years. Yep, you got it in one. A grand total of zero people would have been surprised to learn of the release of levomilnacipran (LVM), the left enantiomer of milnacipran, a few years back. The developers of milnacipran had extra incentive to go down this path as they had been unable to get milnacipran approved for major depression in the USA, leaving it only approved for fibromyalgia, potentially costing hundreds of millions of dollars in lost income. Their strategy appears to have paid off, as they were able to gain approval from the FDA for LVM to be used in major depression.

Like its older sibling (or *parent*, depending on how you view their relationship!), LVM also has the unique ability to inhibit noradrenaline reuptake more potently than serotonin reuptake. In fact, if anything, LVM possesses even more emphasis on noradrenaline. Interestingly however, at higher dosages, LVM's serotonergic effects start to catch up to its effects on noradrenaline, creating a balanced dual reuptake inhibitor at dosages in the upper end of the accepted range. Unfortunately there is no consensus on what size dose would be required to achieve this as there will be significant variation from person to person, as well as variations between *in-vitro* and *in-vivo* tests. For reference, the typical starting dose for LVM is 20mg (so, as usual, I tend to target 10mg instead), an average maintenance dose is 40mg and the official upper dose limit is 120mg.

---

[13] 100% levoamphetamine can be too physically stimulating and therefore unpleasant, so 25% gives just enough of the levo-mediated benefits.

LVM also possesses superior pharmacokinetics, with a longer half-life than the older racemic mixture, which should help prevent any peaks and troughs during the day. However there appears to be some debate as to its metabolism, as some sources state that, like milnacipran, LVM doesn't affect (and isn't affected by) P450 liver enzymes. Whereas other sources indicate that LVM is at least partially metabolised by CYP3A4, along with renal clearance. So perhaps the wisest position to take is to say that there is the chance that LVM could be modestly affected if you are also taking other drugs which are P450 inhibitors.

As LVM is the most potently noradrenal of the SNRIs, its benefits and side-effects relating to noradrenaline can be more pronounced. So first the good news. If you are suffering from a mood disorder which is mediated by low noradrenaline, LVM could potentially be your best option. In addition to the more obvious symptoms such as low energy and low motivation, this type of depression can also be associate with cognitive impairment. As I have mentioned elsewhere, stimulants are effective treatments for ADHD/ADD due largely to their ability to increase noradrenaline levels in the pre-frontal cortex, thereby increasing focus. Low noradrenaline in this part of the brain which is caused by major depression can feature some of these hallmarks of ADHD. Of all the SNRIs, LVM appears to be the most promising first-line option for this scenario. In addition, due to noradrenaline's ability to increase dopamine as a knock-on effect, LVM could also boost mood via this pathway in addition to the serotonin pathway.

So if I were to again apply my two birds with one stone mantra, LVM could be particularly useful in cases where there is both major depression and ADHD present. Particularly considering the resistance which some patients, parents of patients (in the case of adolescent ADHD) and even doctors have in taking stimulants such as methylphenidate. LVM can achieve at least some of the benefits of stimulants but with the key difference being no abuse or addiction potential.

However there is no such thing as a free lunch, so this potent ability to boost noradrenaline comes with some downsides. The probability and intensity of noradrenaline-related side-effects will be higher with LVM than other SNRIs. Of these, sweating, urinary difficulties and nausea appear to be most common.

In addition there are also some cardiovascular side-effects possible which also impact the drug's safety profile. Considering its ability to jack up noradrenaline, it should perhaps come as no surprise to note that some patients can experienced increased blood pressure, elevated heart rate and (usually) minor heart rhythm effects. This means that LVM will be contraindicated if you have certain pre-existing cardiovascular issues. A point I would like to make here which applies to the rest of this book is that you shouldn't assume your doctor or psychiatrist will always bear this in mind. Or perhaps your psychiatrist is unaware of your heart condition as this wasn't communicated properly by your primary doctor or cardiologist.

The good news is that many of these noradrenaline-related side-effects can be managed by alpha-adrenal antagonists such as prazosin (Minipress), or in some cases a beta-blocker such as propranolol (Inderal). Prazosin is particularly effective at improving urinary hesitancy or poor flow.

LVM, like all SNRIs should be used with caution in patients with anxiety disorders. Despite the fact that I have heard many patients report that their anxiety symptoms were improved by LVM or milnacipran, it would be unwise to view it as a first-line treatment for anxiety disorders. Of the anxiety disorders, social anxiety is most likely to benefit from the increase confidence which can emerge as noradrenaline (and then dopamine) levels increase.

As a newer and perhaps more obscure SNRI, milnacipran and LVM are both unavailable in certain countries, such as Australia. However Australian fibromyalgia sufferer advocacy groups are pushing for this situation to be remedied, hoping to replicate the success they had in pushing for pregabalin to be covered by the PBS (Australia's national pharmaceutical subsidy program).

Tricyclic Antidepressants (TCAs)

From the 1950's until the release of Prozac, TCAs were the "gold standard" anxiolytic. However they have now been mostly eschewed by doctors in favour of SSRIs due to the incidence of side-effects and the potential for accidental (and, sadly, deliberate) overdose. The main drawback of TCAs are *antimuscarinic* side effects - dry mouth, dry nose, blurry vision, lowered gastrointestinal motility or constipation, urinary retention, cognitive and/or memory impairment, and increased body temperature.

Antimuscarinic effects are caused when a drug antagonises muscarinic acetylcholine receptors. This is a function of how TCAs were discovered and why they generally also act as super-potent antihistamines (the older antihistamines like promethazine are virtually defined by their antimuscarinic effects. TCAs were discovered by accident in the 1950s when researchers were messing around with an antipsychotic known as chlorpromazine (which you may know as Thorazine), and discovered that certain compounds had the unintended effect of making subjects happy! This led to the release of the first TCA, imipramine, in the late 50s.

TCAs are known as *dirty* drugs, which means that they act on a variety of areas in your brain. They are not *specific* to serotonin like an SSRI. This is an important point as I have found may people see the word "dirty" and read this as a fundamentally *bad* thing. Tramadol is also a "dirty" drug by this definition and I have seen similar comments to the same effect on internet sites as justification for avoiding it. However dirty drugs do have inherent drawbacks for the treating physician because they can trigger unintended effects which can make things complicated to manage. This can cause immediate effects which sometimes need to be managed, such as orthostatic hypotension (which is where you get dizzy when you stand up, due to changes in blood pressure), and effects which take longer to manifest, such as weight gain.

Unsurprisingly then, TCAs as a class have some of the most complex pharmacology of any drug class known. Although there is huge variability between individual TCAs, some of their effects include –

- Serotonin reuptake inhibition
- Noradrenaline reuptake inhibition
- NMDA antagonism
- H1 antagonism (antihistamine)
- Serotonin receptor antagonism
- Anticholinergic effects
- Antimuscarinic effects
- Sodium, calcium and potassium channel blocking
- TrkA and TrkB receptor agonism
- Sigma receptor agonism

The most commonly assumed myth I deal with is that TCAs are less effective than SSRIs. This is entirely false. The main difference between TCAs and SSRIs is that SSRIs tend to have fewer (and less troubling) side effects, meaning that a patient is more likely to continue treatment with an SSRI. Another important distinction is that it is possible to overdose on TCAs, whereas overdosing on SSRIs is virtually impossible. This is largely due to the fact that TCAs are *cardiotoxic*, which means that for some people they can cause cardiovascular problems at therapeutic dosages and at a sufficiently high dose, death for anyone, irrespective of their heart health. Because they can act as sodium, calcium and potassium channel blockers, TCAs can impact cardiac rhythms and decrease heart rate variability, one of the key measures of heart health. However it is important to stress that this is mainly at higher doses. At lower dosage levels, such as the dosages used to treat pain or sleeping problems, it is generally thought that there is little likelihood of issues, unless you have a pre-existing heart problem. Even at doses above this, for most people, the benefits far outweigh the risks. Untreated depression or anxiety is a far greater risk to cardiovascular health.

It is also important to note that each TCA differs in its cardiotoxicity, a factor which can guide clinical decisions where there is potential benefit from TCA therapy in patients at particular cardiovascular risk. The largest analysis of its type found that, statistically speaking, dothiepin was associated with the greatest cardiovascular risk, as well as the greatest incidence of seizures. For me, the most unexpected aspect of this analysis was that nortriptyline was found to be *less* toxic than venlafaxine. Considering that SNRIs are favoured for their reduced toxicity compared to TCAs, this was surprising to say the least.

The same analysis also looked a drug-drug interactions. Despite what you may have read, many psychiatrists mix SSRIs with TCAs for a variety of reasons. For example, someone with both severe depression and neuropathic pain may be prescribed a low dose of amitriptyline along with their SSRI. When you think about it, this is quite a rational strategy as long as there are no significant interactions between the two. You forego the antidepressant effects of the TCA (and therefore, most side effects) and retain the painkilling benefits, with the SSRI taking responsibility for treating the depression. However your doctor must also take any drug-drug interactions into account. In particular, if the SSRI is a potent CYP2D6 inhibitor, the TCA could accumulate to toxic levels. The aforementioned study found that while many of these combinations are relatively safe and effective, one combination which should never be used is fluvoxamine + dothiepin, for this very reason.

Despite their side-effects and risks, many experts believe that TCAs are under-prescribed due to the medical community's current obsession with SSRIs, rather than their efficacy as such. This is why you are more likely to be prescribed a TCA by a psychiatrist, as they have a deeper understanding of the scenarios where TCAs may be warranted. As a result, there are many specialists who found TCAs to be much more reliably effective than SSRIs and continue to use them with many of their patients. This state of affairs is probably the way things should be. If you visit your doctor complaining of anxiety problems or depression and you have never taken any medication for this, an SSRI will almost always be a better first option than a TCA. *Why risk the side-effects of a TCA when an SSRI will suffice?* However a visit to a psychiatrist almost always occurs as a consequence of non-response to your doctor's first "generic" attempt at treatment, so the field of possible drugs and drug categories has already typically narrowed by that stage.

One of the other useful aspects of TCAs is that they appear to decrease your body's ability to sense pain by blocking certain pathways your nerves use to transmit painful stimuli. This is the same reason why SNRIs such as duloxetine can be used to treat certain types of pain. As I touched on briefly before, SNRIs could be thought of as "cleaner" TCAs, as they boost noradrenaline and serotonin, but without the myriad other effects seen with TCAs. This is great when SNRI activity is all you need, but less helpful when we are talking about other pharmacological effects which TCAs can mediate.

This is the reason why TCAs are primarily used these days to treat pain disorders such as fibromyalgia and other forms of neuropathic pain. The choice between TCAs and SNRIs largely depends on the individual psychiatrist, other health conditions you may have and whether your pain may be alleviated by one of the TCA actions which occur independent of serotonin or noradrenaline.

Another potential benefit of TCAs is that each TCA has rather distinct effects, compared to SSRIs, which are significantly more alike as a class. So you have TCAs like doxepin which are primarily antihistamines (and therefore potent sleep aids), or TCAs like clomipramine which are more selective for serotonin and TCAs like dothiepin which are more potent noradrenaline boosters. This is useful because, as I explained earlier in the book, not all mood disorders are related to serotonin and dopamine and even cases where these two neurotransmitters are to blame, reuptake inhibition may not be the answer to your prayers. For example, pure antimuscarinic agents, which have no SNRI activity, improve mood due to downstream effects on serotonin, dopamine and noradrenaline.

Despite their limitations (and there are many), TCAs still hold an important place in the treatment of mood disorders. They are at least as effective as SSRIs, and more so in certain types of depression such as melancholic depression and treatment-resistant depression, however there is a greater price to pay in terms of side-effects. Many people have found them to be highly effective in cases where SSRIs have failed. There is a small but vocal group of practitioners who believe that TCAs are significantly more effective that SSRIs and that the popularity of SSRIs is due largely to pharmaceutical company marketing. Whilst I make no claims in terms of general effectiveness, it is certainly true that for *some* people, they are more effective.

Finally, to apply my *two birds with one stone* thinking again, TCAs like amitriptyline and dothiepin could be a potential option when there is both fibromyalgia and a mood disorder, as it may be possible to treat both with a single drug. Or say we look at in purely in terms of symptoms. Say you appeared before a psychiatrist with the following symptoms –

- Depression or anxiety which had not responded to an SSRI
- Fibromyalgia
- Sleeping difficulties

This would create a strong *prima facie* case for the potential use of a TCA. However one issue here would be the depression/anxiety component. The TCA dose required to treat moderate to severe cases would usually be into cardiotoxic territory and considering that side-effects tend to grow more prominent as dosage escalates, you may experience side-effects which outweigh the benefits. However in cases of mild-to-moderate depression with neuropathic pain, the effective dosage can be much lower, avoiding these issues. For example, the lowest amitriptyline dose believed to be effective for depression would be around 75mg, however many fibromyalgia patients find that 10-25mg can be sufficient for pain relief.

Due to the fact that TCAs are not likely to be your first option and would only be favoured over SSRIs in a small minority of cases, I have not dedicated a large amount of time to all the various individual TCAs (of which there are many). In addition, even when TCAs are used, there are only a handful which make up the vast majority of cases, so I have elected to focus on these drugs only.

Also, because of the often dramatic differences between the drugs which make up this class, I have included a section in the Appendix which shows the binding affinities, along with an explanation on how to read information on binding affinities.

Amitriptyline *(Endep, Elavil)*

This is by far the most widely used TCA due to its balanced reuptake inhibition, along with an excellent reputation for treating neuropathic pain and certain types of headaches (particularly tension headaches, which can be the bane of an anxious person's life). Amitriptyline is also an excellent sleep aid at lower dosages, a useful property considering the overlap between mood disorders and sleeping problems.

In general, the dosages used for sleeping problems and neuropathic pain are much lower than the dosages needed to effectively treat mood disorders such as used for depression and anxiety. Pain and sleep-related dosages are usually between 10-50mg, whereas dosages for mood disorders start around 75mg and go up from there.

As amitriptyline is a TCA, with a TCA's associated cardiovascular effects, try to keep your dosage as low as possible. I should point out however that there is no evidence of any adverse effects on cardiovascular function at sub-75mg levels.

Amitriptyline has one of the most complex pharmacological profiles of any antidepressant, affecting a huge range of different systems. For example, amitriptyline is a –

- serotonin reuptake inhibitor
- noradrenaline reuptake inhibitor
- serotonin receptor antagonist
- alpha-adrenal antagonist
- muscarinic acetylcholine antagonist
- antihistamine
- TrKA& TrKb receptor agonist
- NMDA antagonist (or, negative allosteric modulator, to be more accurate)
- sodium, calcium and potassium channel blocker

The majority of these individual effects have already been covered at various points of the book, however there is a new one buried in the above list which is rather interesting and was only discovered in the past few years. As you will recall, one of the hypothesised reasons behind the antidepressant effect of SSRIs is their ability to boost levels of BDNF (*brain-derived neurotrophic factor*), one of your brain's "fertilisers" which helps you to grow new brain cells through neurogenesis. This activity is particularly concentrated in the hippocampus, which is usually shrunken after a period of chronic stress, high-anxiety or major depression. If you think of BDNF as a kind of neurotransmitter-like "key", it triggers this process of neurogenesis by activating TrKA (*tropomyosine receptor kinase A*, for those of you who need a hobby) receptors.

However in addition, there is another related neuropeptide which also plays a vital role in maintaining the health of your brain at the cellular level – NGF (*nerve-growth factor*). While BDNF is the current "poster child" for neuroplasticity, NGF is no slouch, underpinning or modulating a huge number of beneficial processes such as –

- The repair of *myelin*, the fatty sheath which protects neurons by providing a protective cover for individual *axons*, the tree-like structures which grow out of neurons to enable them to send signals to other neurons. To give you a sense of how important myelin is for your brain, the neurodegenerative condition multiple sclerosis (MS) is caused by damaged myelin.
- Reducing damage to neurons, along with supporting their repair and regeneration. Again, if you want to get a sense of how important this is, Alzheimer's disease is associated with deficient NGF activity
- Reducing neural inflammation

So it's not surprising to learn that impaired NGF function has been associated with not only the above neurodegenerative diseases, but also a wide range of conditions such as depression, schizophrenia and autism.

While BDNF exerts its effects by activating TrKA receptors, NGF activates TrKB receptors. So I was astounded to read a paper published in 2009/10 in which the authors demonstrated that amitriptyline functions as an agonist of both TrKA and TrKB, effectively acting as a "proxy" for BDNF and NGF. Recall that SSRIs are believed to work in part due to their ability to increase levels of BDNF as an indirect effect. Amitriptyline rolls its sleeves up and takes it upon itself to do the job itself!

This US National Institutes of Health-funded study, which was conducted at the *Emory University School of Medicine* and published in the journal *Chemistry & Biology*, found that can amitriptyline can *"impersonate the brain's own growth factors"* and therefore can *"directly stimulate molecules that help neurons grow and resist toxins"*. The research team also studied other TCAs, including imipramine, which is closely related, however only amitriptyline was able to *"duplicate NGF's ability to stimulate neurons to send out neurites, small projections thought to be the beginnings of connections to other neurons."*

This study was not only interesting due to its success in elucidating a new mechanism by which amitriptyline treats mood disorders. It also created the groundwork for future research into TrK receptors. Only recently have researchers discovered the importance of TrKB receptors in the efficacy of antidepressants. Recent research appears to show that when you create TrKB *knockout* mice (which are genetically engineering to lack TrKB receptors), antidepressants won't work when the mice are put into situations which typically induce depression-like states[14]. This particular study demonstrated that amitriptyline's antidepressant effects were

---

[14] Yes, I know, animals are made to suffer awfully in the name of science. There is probably an entire book I could write on the ethical dilemmas involved in making animals suffer to hopefully alleviate our own. I read this stuff every day and I don't think I will ever desensitise enough for it not to affect me.

dependent on TrKB but not TrKA, as TrKA knockout mice were still able to get antidepressant effects from the drug.

This is not to say that TrKA has no relevance to mood disorders or neuroplasticity. However clearly TrKA seems to have a more direct link to mood. This research could provide a springboard for future advances in the treatment of mood disorders. If drug companies can develop a more selective or "cleaner" version of amitriptyline which activates TrK receptors and leaves the other stuff (like muscarinic acetylcholine receptors or sodium, calcium and potassium channels) alone, we may be on to something quite exciting. For example, in addition to NGF and BDNF, there is another neurotrophic factor known as VEGF (*vascular endothelial growth factor*) which may also fill in another missing piece of the overall puzzle. As I covered in detail in Jump Start, one of the benefits of physical exercise is that it exerts antidepressant effects through a range of mechanisms, including its ability to boost BDNF. However in researching this book, I also discovered that exercise boosts VEGF, which in turn accelerates neurogenesis.

Before you race off to your home laboratory to start developing a drug which boosts VEGF, there is another factor to consider. VEGF also helps to build blood vessels, which is why it has been a target of certain anti-cancer drugs. By blocking VEGF, you inhibit the tumour's ability to grow, as a malignant tumour's rapid growth must be supported by equally rapid growth of blood vessels. So theoretically (and by theoretically, I mean – I am literally guessing, as I have no background in oncology) a drug which increased VEGF could potentially be dangerous if you happened to have a tumour somewhere in your body. Did I mention that research into mood disorders can be rather complicated?

This issue of amitriptyline's messy pharmacology is important. I want to make sure that the above story regarding its TrK activity doesn't make amitriptyline out to be a miracle drug. It isn't for most people. For those using amitriptyline for pain relief at 10-25mg, some see immense benefits, others none. And some experience such intolerable side-effects at 25mg, the concept of taking 200mg or more for depression would seem incomprehensible. This is a drug which can cause all the moisture in their mouth to take a leave of absence, or make a simple visit to the bathroom take ten-times as long due to difficulty urinating, or cause significant weight gain. However this is also a drug, which for a small sub-set of people, can pull them out of a lifelong, deep, dark hole. Hit Google and type in "amitriptyline user reviews" if you would like to get a sense of the dramatic variation in effects from person to person.

As with most SSRIs, amitriptyline is primarily metabolised by CYP2D6 (and to a lesser extent, CYP2C19), so concomitantly taking a drug which inhibits these enzymes, or in people who are CYP2D6 ultra-metabolisers or poor metabolisers, amitriptyline is not recommended. TCAs are not to be trifled with. If you are a CYP2D6 ultra-metaboliser or poor metaboliser taking an SSRI, there is little risk posed. However if you cannot clear amitriptyline from your system, it can pose certain risks. Alternatively, if your body is too efficient at clearing the drug, you won't be able to see therapeutic effects. The problem with amitriptyline and other TCAs is that the therapeutic window is quite narrow. The difference between "only just working" and "overdose/death" is smaller than other drugs used to treat mood disorders.

Again, this is where an experienced psychiatrist is invaluable. They will know what a safe and sensible dosage would be to start off, whereupon you can gradually taper upwards, at a slow enough speed that you will be able see the effects as they manifest, making the probability of an overshoot unlikely.

Finally, I wanted to briefly address something I only discovered in the process of researching this book. As I will cover later in the section on MAOIs, one of the golden rules of antidepressant therapy is that MAOIs should never be combined with other serotonergic drugs due to the risk of serotonin syndrome, which is a potentially fatal condition. However, this also gives researchers a way to investigate whether a particular drug increases serotonin in any meaningful way. If, in experiments or via real world case studies, a drug is combined with a MAOI and no serotonin toxicity develops, it is probably not serotonergic to any great extent. This is important as often our understanding of the pharmacology of antidepressants is based on in-vitro binding studies. Sometimes a drug can appear to do one thing in a test tube and have completely different effects in the human body.

This issue of serotonin toxicity when combining a drug with a MAOI is why many experts dispute the ability of mirtazapine (which I will cover later in the book) to affect serotonin in any noticeable way. However what I didn't know was that amitriptyline also "failed" this test in the large scale review of TCAs I mentioned earlier. In contrast, clomipramine elicits dangerous serotonin toxicity when combined with a MAOI.

For me, there are two main takeaways from this. Firstly, if serotonin is your problem, amitriptyline is unlikely to be a good candidate. Secondly, this again reinforces a repeating theme throughout this book – that expert care is required when establishing your treatment protocol – especially when more than one drug is combined. In a hypothetical (albeit highly unlikely) scenario where you are taking a MAOI for depression and your doctor decides to add a TCA for neuropathic pain[15], a choice between say, amitriptyline and clomipramine, could be the difference between life or death.

---

[15] I should point out that any doctor who adds a TCA to a MAOI (particularly a GP/primary care physician) should have their right to practice medicine

Clomipramine *(Anafranil)*

There is, quite rightly, much debate as to the link between low serotonin and mood disorders. Depending on the context, boosting dopamine or noradrenaline can alleviate depression, which is all the more strange when you realise that in many cases, boosting dopamine can actually *suppress* serotonin. Or, to look at it from a different angle, if you were foolhardy or of a particular inclination, snorting cocaine[16] (which almost exclusively sends dopamine through the roof), would in most cases, almost miraculously "cure" your depression almost immediately (lasting for about 30 minutes before you then endured a day or so of feeling dramatically worse than you did before). Clearly serotonin is accorded no particular exclusivity in terms of its ability to make you "happy".

However, when we are talking about the myriad anxiety disorders which afflict us, a different picture emerges. More serotonin floating around in your synapses can make *some* people less depressed, however it tends to make *almost everyone* less anxious. For essentially all anxiety disorders except social anxiety (which, depending on the person, can also have a dopamine/noradrenaline component), your search for the most effective drug must almost always be centred on serotonin. That is why the most serotonergic of all SSRIs (paroxetine) has the most compelling evidence in the treatment of moderate to severe anxiety and why clomipramine is the TCA doctors usually turn to in similar situations.

Clomipramine is by far the single most potent serotonergic TCA available. If you have severe anxiety caused by low levels of serotonin and you are able to tolerate the side-effects, clomipramine can sometimes have life-changing effects when all else has failed.

In particular, many clinicians are of the opinion that clomipramine is the single most effective treatment for obsessive compulsive disorder (OCD). As I mentioned earlier, OCD tends to require powerful serotonergic drugs or drugs at dosages far exceeding what is required for other mood disorders. As a result, clomipramine is rarely used as a first or second-line treatment for depression. As a TCA, with all of the usual downsides of TCAs, it would be pointless for someone with "garden variety" depression to put up with the side-effects when in all likelihood an SSRI would suffice. That doesn't mean that clomipramine doesn't treat depression, however it would need to be depression which is at the upper end of the severity-scale for it to be worthwhile.

In addition to OCD, clomipramine is also believed to be one of the most effective medications for moderate-to-severe panic disorder, often reducing the frequency and severity of panic attacks within 2 weeks of beginning treatment.

---

[16] This goes without saying however I just wanted to mention what a terrible idea this would be – particularly for someone who has made it this far through a book on antidepressants.

Whilst clomipramine is undeniably effective for OCD and panic disorder, most doctors will want to try an SSRI such as fluvoxamine or paroxetine first because most trials show that these newer SSRIs are roughly as effective in clinical trials, but with less side-effects. However this is far from written in stone. For example, I have talked to psychopharmacologists with decades of experience who immediately turn to clomipramine when faced with a patient at the severe end of the scale, irrespective of whether the problem is mood or anxiety. Their rationale is understandable. Imagine you were in their shoes and you had treated say, 200 patients for severe mood disorders over the course of your career. If, in 150 of those cases you had started with an SSRI which didn't work, before switching to clomipramine, which did, you would probably just skip the SSRI and go straight to clomipramine.

It is important to realise that, when a doctor is faced with a patient who is severely depressed, self-harm will always figure prominently in their thinking. If a patient is severely depressed (and particularly if there is also suicidal ideation), they might not have the luxury of trial and error, trying to find a drug with a good trade-off between efficacy and side-effects. So in these cases, many may make an informed decision to "pull out the big guns" and start with clomipramine.

In terms of side-effects, clomipramine is associated with the typical TCA effects such as dry mouth, constipation and cardiovascular effects. However clomipramine is without equal regarding several of these. Firstly, clomipramine has a significantly higher seizure risk than other antidepressants (perhaps with the exception of bupropion, which I will cover later). There are certain drugs which lower the "seizure threshold", which is the threshold of certain neurological or neurochemical activity sufficient to trigger a seizure. In addition to clomipramine and bupropion, tramadol is another drug notorious for lowering this threshold. The problem with combining two drugs which lower the threshold is that the effects can be additive, lowering the threshold to a level where there would be a distinct possibility of a seizure being triggered. If this happened to you, the first you would probably know about it would be when you wake up in hospital. That is *if* you wake up. This is not something to take chances with, so combining multiple drugs like this should only be done with great care, under the close eye of an experienced psychiatrist.

The other side-effect where clomipramine punches above its weight is sexual dysfunction. Considering the close correlation between high serotonin and sexual dysfunction, it should come as no surprise to learn that clomipramine is particularly associated with sexual dysfunction.

Imipramine & Desipramine *(Tofranil, Norpramin)*

As touched on before, imipramine was the very first TCA, essentially discovered by accident a half a century ago. Just like the process of refinement which followed the release of the first SSRI, fluoxetine, leading to more targeted drugs like escitalopram, imipramine sparked a flurry of research which led to follow-up TCAs such as amitriptyline. And as you could probably imagine, targeted research was able to generate improvements over an accidental, serendipitously discovered imipramine. That's not to say that imipramine is ineffective. It is still considered the "gold standard" antidepressant against which all other options are measured. For so much research, a drug will regularly be compared to imipramine and placebo. However it is also important to highlight that "gold standard" sometimes implies "the best". However in this case it is better to think of imipramine's value as "1.0", so if a new drug is twice as effective as imipramine, it would be "2.0". Opioids are measured in a similar way, with morphine as the gold-standard baseline above or below which will sit other opioids in terms of potency.

My issue with imipramine is that it occupies a kind of middle-ground where it performs acceptably in each of the mechanisms that antidepressants are assessed for (serotonin reuptake, noradrenaline reuptake etc.), yet isn't "best in class" for any. Clomipramine is more serotonergic, amitriptyline is better for pain and doxepin is better for sleep. When you or your doctor are looking for the most effective option, you will no doubt be using a range of criteria. Armed with this criteria I generally struggle to come up with a scenario where imipramine would be my first candidate.

So its use is now largely confined to situations where the most logical options have been exhausted already. And in these scenarios, there is a small sub-set of the population who just happen to respond to imipramine, for whatever reason, be it pharmacodynamics or pharmacokinetics.

Speaking of pharmacodynamics, imipramine is a fairly strong inhibitor of serotonin reuptake, negligible noradrenaline reuptake, and middle of the road anticholinergic side-effects. However one of its metabolites is desipramine, which has the inverse – negligible serotonin reuptake and strong noradrenaline reuptake. Firstly, this means that you shouldn't base your assessment on the primary effects of imipramine, as you would need to take the effects of desipramine into account.

Secondly, desipramine itself is available as a TCA for cases requiring an emphasis on noradrenaline reuptake.

Doxepin *(Sinequan)*

One of the topics which most surprises those I talk to, is the relationship of antidepressants with antihistamines. Most people imagine these two drug types as being unrelated, finding it hard to draw the connection between a drug which stops you from sneezing during hay fever season and a drug which makes you "happier". Perhaps in the example of TCAs, which also function as antihistamines, this becomes a little easier to understand. However you may be shocked to learn that Prozac was developed from diphenhydramine, an antihistamine better known in most places as Benadryl. And diphenhydramine is itself partly an SSRI, something I am sure would horrify those who consider SSRIs as "toxic", seeing as they have probably been giving it to their children when they have had a cold or to treat their hay fever. Oh, and while I mention it, another little known piece of important information is that you should avoid diphenhydramine if you are taking an SSRI, due to a potential (yet, a little overstated) risk of serotonin toxicity.

Imagine inside your brain there are small buttons to push to cause certain effects. So there is a "serotonin reuptake" button, a "noradrenaline reuptake" button and so on. In this figurative example, the "antihistamine" button is located right next to the buttons associated with treating mood disorders. So, when you press one of these tiny buttons using a large "finger", it is difficult to press one without also pressing the other, like I often do when trying to type a message on my iPhone's tiny LCD keyboard.

This means that sometimes a drug is placed in either the "antihistamine" category or the "antidepressant" category for reasons which are unclear. There is probably a parallel universe where diphenhydramine is an antidepressant and mirtazapine (which I am yet to cover) is an antihistamine. Similarly, I can't help but think the decision to label doxepin as an antidepressant is rather arbitrary. Diphenhydramine, mirtazapine and doxepin all have very similar potency as antihistamines, being essentially the strongest currently available. So surely the decision to call doxepin an antidepressant must be based on its serotonin and/or noradrenaline reuptake, right?

Strangely, no. Doxepin's serotonin reuptake is only marginally more potent than diphenhydramine's and its noradrenaline reuptake is even weaker than its serotonergic effects. In fact, aside from its H1 antihistamine effects, doxepin doesn't really do much at all. This may provide an explanation as to why, when you type "doxepin anti" into Google, it autocompletes with "antihistamine" *before* "antidepressant".

It is for this reason that doxepin is mostly used as a sleep aid due to its super-potent H1 effects. However even this provides no satisfactory reason why a doctor would prescribe it. Mirtazapine is a lot "cleaner" (with none of the TCA-related cardiotoxicity and less anticholinergic activity) and diphenhydramine is easier to obtain, available OTC from most pharmacies. So if someone with major depression or an anxiety disorder asked for my input, I could not in good conscience send them away with a recommendation to turn to doxepin with any expectation of serotonergic or noradrenergic benefits.

At a stretch, I guess I could go as far as saying that mild anxiety disorders can sometimes be helped by antihistamines, due to their general sedating properties. So if someone had mild anxiety along with sleep disturbances and mirtazapine was out of the question for whatever reason, doxepin could potentially help. However what little antidepressant effects doxepin has, should be considered as a "bonus extra" on top of its antihistamine properties.

Dosulepin/Dothiepin[17] (Dothep, Prothiaden)

Dothiepin is yet another TCA with fairly generic pharmacology, essentially having serotonergic and noradrenergic activity which is half that of amitriptyline. So, variations in how different people metabolise dothiepin and amitriptyline aside, it could be considered as a *milder* amitriptyline.

These days dothiepin is rarely used specifically for depression or anxiety, its use mainly limited to neuropathic pain conditions such as fibromyalgia. Strangely, last time I checked it wasn't available at all in the US, with most use concentrated in the UK and Australia.

It is considered one of the milder TCAs, so accordingly, some doctors use it for mild depression or anxiety. However, if you have mild depression or anxiety, I would usually contend that you would be better off looking at non-drug treatments. The side-effects of TCAs often create a poor trade-off at the best of times, so it seems pointless to use a TCA like dothiepin for cases where drugs may not even be needed.

However in more serious cases, it could be a potential to amitriptyline if, for whatever reason, amitriptyline doesn't agree with you. Of the various mood disorders, dothiepin seems to work best for anxiety-related issues. In particular, due to its pain-relieving properties, fibromyalgia with concomitant anxiety tends to be the most common scenario under which it would be used. This often involves a dosage around 25mg and occasionally as high as 75mg (which is usually given in 3 doses, spread evenly throughout the day).

However, moderate-to-severe depression or OCD requires dosages up around 200mg. There is some research which suggests that dothiepin is the most cardiotoxic TCA at these higher dosages (which were fairly standard when TCAs were a mainstay of depression treatment before SSRIs arrive on the scene), so except in the rarest of cases, other options would be preferable. I should say however that there is little evidence to suggest cardiotoxicity at the lower, pain-related dosages.

Otherwise, dothiepin is associated with the same upsides and downsides as other TCAs, such as antihistamine-mediated sedation and dry mouth. However one, more unusual side-effect which I have seen on multiple occasions is photosensitivity. Patients often start dothiepin and then notice that they are getting sunburnt after only brief sun exposure. This is particularly an issue in Australia, parts of which feel like they are located only miles from the sun.

---

[17] Dosulepin was renamed dothiepin in 1998. I have no idea why and have never been sufficiently interested to find out.

With the current popularity of SSRIs, backed up by TCAs for harder to treat cases, MAOIs have largely become a drug of a bygone era due to their side-effects and hotly-debated dietary risks. However contrary to expectations, MAOIs are still widely used for severe types of depression such as treatment resistant depression or *melancholic* forms.

However, to the extent that modern psychopharmacology is able to alleviate the suffering of millions (albeit imperfectly, still to this day) by boosting serotonin and other monoamines, we owe MAOIs a debt of gratitude. MAOIs first showed us the link between monoamines and depression. Like TCAs and arguably, like SSRIs, the discovery of the first MAOI was serendipitous.

Back in the 1950s, researchers studying a tuberculosis drug called *isoniazid* noticed that it had the rather unusual side-effect of making depressed patients less depressed. Soon after, this led to the development of the first MAOI (iproniazid), which was a modified version of isoniazid. Unfortunately, iproniazid was associated with high rates of hepatitis, so was taken off the market in most countries (except, intriguingly, France[18]). However this was followed by the development of *phenelzine* and *tranylcypromine*, drugs which remain in (limited) use today.

As mentioned earlier, MAOIs act by preventing an enzyme called *monoamine oxidase* from breaking up (or *deaminating*) monoamines such as serotonin, dopamine & noradrenaline. Normally, this enzyme breaks down these three monoamines to use for "recycling", so by preventing this, they are able to remain in the synapse for longer, leading to increased levels.

There are two types (isoforms) of MAO: *MAO-A* and *MAO-B*.

MAO-A breaks down serotonin, noradrenaline, dopamine and tyramine (it is the tyramine which creates the dietary challenges I will mention in a moment). MAO-B only breaks down dopamine. Depending on which of these two forms are affected by a given MAOI, the effects and indeed the effectiveness, will be different.

MAOIs are rarely used these days due to their undesirable side-effect profile and (potential) safety issues. While someone is taking a MAOI, they must usually conform to inconvenient dietary restrictions such as no red wine or aged cheeses, because the tyramine in these foods can sometimes cause a life-threatening blood pressure issue which can be fatal. Normally, when we consume food with tyramine, it triggers the release of noradrenaline which is then mopped up by MAO-A. However when MAO-A is suppressed, noradrenaline can spike to dangerous levels, causing a hypertensive crisis.

---

[18] Those whacky continental Europeans!

However, the experienced psychopharmacologists I talked to for this book have often had great results with MAOIs when all else failed. This is why they are typically reserved for treatment resistant depression (TRD). Another common piece of feedback I get from experts is that the risks associated with MAOIs are overstated. This is important to bear in mind. Many patients are successfully using MAOIs with few dietary restrictions. For example, in general, only a small number of aged cheeses cause issues. The cheese you most likely consume in your daily diet, such as non-aged cheddar or processed cheese, are usually fine. And not every bottle of wine is high in tyramine. That said, if it were me, I don't think I would want to bet my life on a wine-maker's ability to accurately measure the tyramine content of their product. I would probably stick to less-risky forms of alcohol. Better yet, if I was sufficiently unwell to warrant a MAOI, I would probably stay away from alcohol altogether, considering the havoc it plays with neurotransmitters.

You may find that you can tolerated MAOIs safely with little disruption to your typical dietary habits. However if in doubt, talk to your doctor (and in this case, I mean psychiatrist – you should not assume that your doctor is experienced in guiding patients through MAOI therapy).

MAOIs are kind of like your "In case of emergency break glass" backup option when all else fails. You might not need them. You might not be able to tolerate them. However when they work, they *really* work. If you do a bit of internet searching for user experiences you will find countless stories of MAOIs being life changing, just when all hope had been lost.

You should hope you will never need them, but you may be extremely grateful for their potency if you do.

In general, MAOIs are not usually used to treat anxiety disorders except in rare, often severe, cases. Due to their ability to potently boost noradrenaline and dopamine they can be quite stimulating, which is often useful for depression but less so for anxiety. However there are exceptions, which I will cover in a moment.

After MAOIs, the next option down the list of potential treatments would be electroconvulsive therapy (ECT) – another treatment which would really only be utilised in desperate circumstances such as severe, intractable depression. However again this is specific to depression. It is rare to see an anxiety disorder which doesn't respond to *any* drug. Despite their addictiveness and other issues, I haven't seen many cases where benzodiazepines didn't reduce anxiety, and even if they didn't, you would still have barbiturates as a backup in severe cases. ECT and MAOIs are not typically needed for severe anxiety.

MAOIs are widely considered to be the most powerful antidepressants available and if the side-effect profile was better, MAOIs would be the first line pharmacological treatment for depression. One thing I have seen over and over when scouring PubMed is the following statement –

"Drug X is as effective as TCAs and SSRIs, but less effective than MAOIs"

However this high degree of potency is the reason why MAOIs have a particularly strict list of drugs you cannot be taking at the same time, due to the risk of serotonin syndrome. Essentially, anything which is even vaguely serotonergic is proscribed. From SSRIs and TCAs (which should come as no surprise) all the way down to the amino acid l-tryptophan, which as you will recall is the building blocks for serotonin. One thing you will probably realise if you trial more than one antidepressant is that most of the drugs which we are warned will cause serotonin toxicity are closer to "guidelines" than strict rules. I have dealt with many people whose psychiatrist has them on combinations such as tramadol + SSRIs, with no issues. Most of the time, combinations like these only cause issues for a small subset of patients or patients taking high dosages of both. As long as your psychiatrist knows what you are combining, they will usually know what is and isn't safe.

However there is no such leeway with MAOIs. Not only is their potency an issue, due to the way they work, if serotonin spikes to dangerous levels, your brain has no way to clear it, as MAO has been blocked.

I want to avoid spending too much time on the older, first generation MAOIs. Not because they are ineffective. On the contrary, they may be the most effective antidepressants available. My rationale is that if you need the help of these drugs, not only is their use a little more complicated due to interactions and side-effects, by definition you will probably be in need of some individual, one-on-one therapy with an expert psychopharmacologist. I am conscious of the fact that I want this book to be of practical use, however this is one small corner of the overall picture where I fear I cannot be of much help.

However what I can do is briefly mention the two MAOIs which will most likely be used, if it is determined that they will be your best option.

First-generation irreversible MAOIs

By far the most commonly prescribed MAOIs are Phenelzine (Nardil) and Tranylcypromine (Parnate). Both of these drugs operate in roughly the same way, however Nardil is slightly more potent at inhibiting MAO-A, whereas Parnate has a (comparatively) stronger action inhibiting MAO-B. While both can be extremely effective and which one is better depends on the individual, Parnate's dopamine-boosting effects can make people so "happy" that they can almost feel high. Interestingly, there has been recent research which appears to show that the reason why tobacco smoking is so pleasurable is actually only weakly related to nicotine. After all, you can't chew nicotine gum and get high. In fact, it appears that tobacco's pleasurable aspects come from its activity as a MAOI, with effects concentrated on MAO-B, giving smokers a nice dopamine boost. So, whilst I strongly urge you to not suddenly take up smoking, if you are a current or past smoker and remember the feeling you first got from smoking, this may roughly approximate the general "flavour" of a MAOI.

Reversible versus irreversible MAOIs

As you could probably imagine, with the discovery of the first generation MAOIs, with their safety risks due to the tyramine effect, it was only natural that research would be dedicated to developing safer MAOIs. Eventually it was discovered that the problem was the fact that the early MAOIs were irreversible. Once the drug attached to the MAO, it clung on for dear life and never let go. Imagine MAO having a "lock" like the serotonin or dopamine receptors I mentioned earlier. The irreversible MAOIs are like super-glue being poured into the lock. You then need to wait for the locksmith to come out with new MAO locks, which takes time. Meanwhile, if you ingested tyramine, the MAO would be out of action, unable to deal with the spike in noradrenaline.

This led to the development of reversible MAOIs (or officially – *reversible inhibitors of monoamine oxidase* – RIMAs) which mitigated this issue. In the event of a tyramine effect, a RIMA gets dislodged from the MAO, bring it back into service, whereupon it starts "kicking ass and taking names", dealing with the noradrenaline riff-raff. [19]

---

[19] I have always imagined it would look like one of those movies where the "superhero/wizard/" gets back their trusty "staff/large hammer/spinach" just in time to "save the day". I know what you're thinking. I may need a hobby.

Moclobemide (*Aurorix*)

First, a warning. I initially want to address something which is a more general point on the availability of certain drugs. If you have no interest in this particular topic, please skip ahead a few paragraphs.

If ever you needed further confirmation that the world of Big Pharma and the US FDA makes no sense whatsoever, let me present moclobemide as *Exhibit A*. You see, RIMAs were developed as a safer alternative to MAOIs, due to the risks associated with the older irreversible MAOIs. Perhaps you might have expected the US health authorities to yank the old MAOIs off the shelves (which, by the way, I wouldn't support, considering the value they still have) and have them replaced by RIMAs like moclobemide quick-smart. On the contrary, it is the older MAOIs which are still available and it is moclobemide which isn't even available in the US! When I looked into the reason for this while researching this book, beyond the Wikipedia entry which states

> *"Due to a lack of financial incentive, such as the costs of conducting the necessary trials to gain approval, moclobemide is unavailable in the USA pharmaceutical market."*

Whilst I am sure that there is more to the story than what is public knows, I found this to be a curious state of affairs, as moclobemide is widely used throughout the world, including Australia and the UK. These older drugs, some of which have liver toxicity issues, others with bad side-effects and all with the common tyramine issue are potentially being prescribed to certain people whose quality of life is then impacted. Also, I found the reference to the cost of conducting trials to be rather eyebrow-raising. Moclobemide was developed in Switzerland in 1972 so is long off-patent as far as I know. And it is so long ago, I have struggled to find out why it was never released in the US when it still had patent protection. As someone who believes that people have a right to access the best possible treatment, this raises a few troubling questions, like -

- Many, many drugs each year are developed by small companies such as biotech start-ups, before beginning the process of FDA-approval. Whoever developed moclobemide (even this is murky, with references pointing to an entity or researcher called Wyss, based out of Basel), they would have known that the "big game in town" is the US market and that the FDA-approval process would take time and money. So I am curious why this never occurred.
- Today, the giant Swiss pharma Hoffmann-La Roche markets moclobemide around the world. This is a company who could easily afford to go through the process of approval.
- However perhaps they don't because any generic drug maker could ride in on their coat tails after approval.

- Lastly, this was the last in a series of "coincidences" I noticed when researching this book. Almost every drug I saw which was not available in the US, or was not approved for a major indication such as depression, was owned by a foreign pharmaceutical company

I am certainly not advocating certain drugs being exempt from the FDA approval process, as this is an incredibly important step. In fact, I would hazard a guess that the rest of the world benefits from the FDA-approval process. Because the US market is so huge, the FDA can demand drug companies conduct expensive trials – the results of which are used to guide lawmakers in other countries. Perhaps a more pragmatic compromise in cases like this could be for the developer to gain patent-holder rights for the standard number of years. This would give these drug companies enough of a rationale to submit to the FDA process.

At the end of the day, all I care about is that people around the world can get access to safe, effective drugs which could be the difference between life and death in some cases. Whether this refers to people in third-world countries getting access to anti-malarial drugs or a depressed person in the US who responds to MAOIs but can't tolerate the side-effects, the motivation is similar.

/end rant

OK, now that I have that off my chest, let's return to moclobemide in the context of mood disorders.

The first thing I need to do however is to ensure that the above (and, admittedly, rather tangential) point on the lack of US market availability doesn't overplay the importance or effectiveness of moclobemide. While there is plenty of research data to suggest that moclobemide can be as effective as SSRIs and TCAs, there is still a rather large gulf between this group of drugs and the older MAOIs. To convey this situation in quantitative or numerical terms, in my estimation, moclobemide is probably 30-40% less effective than older MAOIs. However on the flip-side, moclobemide's side-effects are probably 80-90% less prominent, plus there is only a very small risk with the tyramine effect.

If you have severe, debilitating and disabling depression, the above numbers probably say *I am happy to put up with the side-effects in return for that 30-40% efficacy advantage*. However if you are more at the moderate end of the spectrum, or you responded to an older MAOI but couldn't tolerate the side-effects, moclobemide starts to look pretty attractive.

Moclobemide is a useful alternative to SSRIs, TCAs and older MAOIs, which has some interesting pharmacological effects which make it rather novel. It is a selective, reversible inhibitor of MAO-A, which means it boosts levels of serotonin, noradrenaline and to a slightly lesser extent, dopamine. This makes it useful in a number of cases, like when you have issues with noradrenaline and dopamine, as well as serotonin, making SSRIs less appropriate. Or when you have the same issue, but TCAs are either not allowed (due to cardiovascular problems) or the side-effects are too bad.

Chronic treatment of moclobemide at sufficient dosages has also been shown to trigger down-regulation of beta-adrenoceptors (β-adrenergic receptors). More broadly, this process, whereby there is less activation of beta-adrenergic receptors, is another hypothesized mechanism behind the efficacy of antidepressants therapy over time. As it is fairly easy to measure, this has therefore been proposed as a future diagnostic tool, such as when your doctor wants to evaluate your non-subjective response to a drug. Moclobemide appears to be particularly effective at this.

One of the most attractive aspects of moclobemide are its unique effects (among most other antidepressants) on testosterone. While SSRIs and TCAs are associated with sexual dysfunction (primarily due to the effects on prolactin and dopamine), moclobemide can be pro-sexual, due to its rather surprising ability to dramatically boost testosterone and perhaps also the minor dopamine bump. A common source of frustration for doctors who have never experienced antidepressant-related sexual dysfunction is when a patient stops therapy due to this reason. There is sometimes an unspoken implication that the patient *"should be grateful that their depression is improving"* and that their complaints regarding libido or erectile dysfunction are *"just being fussy"*.

Firstly, what I will say to this is, wanting to mitigate a significant side-effect such as this is not being fussy. Sure, if you have gone from not getting out of bed for weeks, gripped by severe depression, to feeling "normal" or happy, thanks to a particular drug, and then you tell your doctor you want to quit because it is "ruining your complexion", that might qualify as fussy. However sexual function is often a core piece of our identity, or helps us to feel pleasure. Sexual contact is also a major component of our relationship with our partner. So "not feeling up to it" can trigger feelings of irrational shame, worried that your partner may think less of you[20]. If your drug is causing sexual side-effects, go back to your doctor to discuss your options for managing the issue, either by adding in another drug (such as bupropion or mirtazapine) or by switching drugs.

Another relatively unique aspect of moclobemide is its ability to improve cognitive function, in contrast with many other antidepressants. Particularly TCAs, owing to their anticholinergic/antimuscarinic properties, tend to worsen cognitive function. For most people this is manageable, however for the elderly, older antidepressants can often be disorienting or lead to confused thinking. Due to this property,

---

[20] In 99.99% of cases where there is a loving relationship, I think your partner would happily give up sex if it meant they could have the "old you" back. Sometimes it is easy to forget that your partner is also affected, as it can be difficult to watch someone you love in pain.

moclobemide is even used as a nootropic (cognitive enhancer) by some. I assume this is caused by increases in dopamine and noradrenaline in the prefrontal cortex.

As it boosts serotonin, which quells anxiety, and dopamine, which gives you confidence, of all the various anxiety disorders, moclobemide is particularly suited to social anxiety. It even has some evidence showing it is effective at reducing pain levels in those with fibromyalgia. This could be partly explained by moclobemide's anti-inflammatory properties, which are believed to contribute to its antidepressant effects and could also feasibly be a factor in its ability to reduce pain[21].

Ironically (or at least, unfairly) moclobemide is one of the safest antidepressants available. Of all the major antidepressants, it is probably the most underutilised. That's not to say that it should always be the first thing doctors think of. However when doctors and patients see the word "MAOI", there can be a great deal of resistance due to an unfair rap. It is the pharmacological equivalent of *guilt by association*. I have even heard rumours that this issue played at large part in the reason why no one has invested money into obtaining FDA approval. There may be a sense that it could be a nightmare trying to educate doctors and patients on the differences between moclobemide and old-school irreversible MAOIs.

When I researched each drug in this book, I first spent a lot of time going through clinical trial information. Then I spent a lot of time looking at sites with either user reviews or forum discussions. Whilst all drugs have a range of effects which vary from person to person, moclobemide seemed to have the most dramatic disparity between positive and negative reviews. Those in the positive camp would wax lyrical about the life-changing effects (with some even saying that moclobemide felt almost "recreational"[22]). Those in the negative camp either said it was horrible (in terms of side-effects), or it had no effect whatsoever.

However no drug is risk-free or side-effect free. While being nothing like the irreversible MAOIs, moclobemide still has a small tyramine effect which you may need to bear in mind. It is also associated with the "classic" antidepressant side effects including dry mouth, constipation and nausea – particularly at start-up. However these usually settle down over time. Another possibility at start-up is some transient insomnia, as it can be a little activating to start.

Like most antidepressants, the main danger associated with moclobemide is serotonin syndrome, if you combine it with other serotonergic agents such as SSRIs. This means that you also need to take care when switching to and from moclobemide. Your doctor will need to provide guidance on a tapering plan. While you can just jump from SSRI to similar drugs without tapering, more care must be taken with moclobemide. It has managed to shake off much of its heritage however

---

[21] I should point out that the link between inflammation and fibromyalgia is a complicated one. Some cases appear to involve elevated biomarkers for inflammation, whereas others don't.

[22] Yes I know what you just thought. Don't even think about it!

there are some classic MAOI-type complications which remain. Please check all possible drug interactions with your doctor. This includes drugs which, despite appearing benign, could be problematic. For example, the common heartburn/ulcer drug cimetidine (Tagamet) can increase levels of moclobemide by *double*, which is a significant change that could be a recipe for problems.

Meanwhile, let's hope the current situation changes so that American citizens can get access to this drug.

Selegiline *(Deprenyl, Emsam)*

Now that we have looked at the main reversible inhibitor of MAO-A, let's look at a selective, reversible inhibitor of MAO-B.

Due to its selectivity for MAO-B (and therefore, dopamine) selegiline is primarily used to treat Parkinson's disease, however it is also used as an antidepressant. In fact, in 2006 a transdermal patch (Emsam) was approved by the FDA for the specific treatment of major depression. The patch, which, like nicotine patches, enables you to absorb the drug through the skin, bit by bit over a 24 hour period, before the patch is changed for a new one. The patch not only enables you to keep levels of selegiline stable in your system, it bypasses the drug's poor oral absorption.

Selegiline is a cytochrome P450 enzyme inhibitor, however CYP2A6 is the only isoform affected. Compared to CYP2D6, CYP2A6 metabolises few drugs and therefore selegiline creates fewer complications that drugs like fluoxetine. Probably the only "common" drug affected by this is nicotine

One thing that often scares people about selegiline is that it is a distant cousin of methamphetamine, however it shares few of the effects of methamphetamine and is in no way "recreational". Although I am sure if I searched forums like Bluelight, there will be some "shallow end of the gene pool" types who try to get high off selegiline. In effect, selegiline has as much in common with meth as Immodium (loperamide) does with morphine[23]. This very rudimentary distinction has even been lost on certain governments, such as Japan's, where selegiline is strictly controlled due to the meth-link. One thing which doesn't help the situation is the fact that when you metabolise selegiline, an insignificant amount of methamphetamine is produced. It is for this reason that you may need to inform the tester if your company has random drug tests, in case selegiline causes a false-positive for meth.

The irony here is that selegiline is actually a powerful neurotrophic/neuroprotective agent which can be used to gradually "heal" the brain of a recovering meth addict. In the short terms, selegiline can also help to restore the dopamine lost to the meth high.

This is more than a little ironic when you realise that selegiline is not only safe, effective and non-addictive, it is also neuroprotective, helping to prevent Parkinsonian symptoms in animal trials.

Considering its pharmacology, I guess it goes without saying that it is best-suited to those whose mood issues are related to a lack of dopamine. If you have atypical depression, or your symptoms involve a lack of energy, motivation or you no longer

---

[23] This is another one which surprises people. Immodium is an opioid, however it has been designed not to cross the blood brain barrier, so has no euphoric properties.

derive pleasure from doing the things you love, selegiline could be an option worth discussing with your doctor.

Atypical Antidepressants

"Atypical antidepressants" is really just the drug companies' way of saying "everything else", as the drugs in this category have little in common, mostly working in completely different ways. However this isn't the same situation as when you were a kid at school playing sport where each captain would choose their players and get to the last batch of kids who couldn't play sport very well. The following drugs are often just as effective as SSRIs, however due to their disparate range of actions, they are sometimes the only drug which works in that particular way. So they just get lumped in the rather awkward "atypical" category.

Bupropion *(Wellbutrin, Zyban)*

Bupropion is often confusing for doctors and patients alike, as in many countries it is primarily used to help people quit smoking. This is particularly the case here in Australia where it is not officially recognised as an antidepressant. So if you are a smoker (who is otherwise happy) and you visit your doctor asking for help to quit smoking, it is relatively easy to walk out with a government-subsidised script for bupropion. If you are seriously depressed and visit the same doctor, they won't typically even consider bupropion as an option. I tried this out myself last time I visited my own GP, asking him how often he has prescribed bupropion for depression. He was unaware that bupropion was used as an antidepressant in the USA.

This is a shame, as bupropion fills a hole in the pharmacological arsenal we have for treating depression. Short of resorting to stimulants like methylphenidate, there are no options for inhibiting the reuptake of dopamine (aside from sertraline's modest abilities in this area). Bupropion's relatively unique mechanism of action amongst antidepressants makes it a useful option for those have not responded to SSRIs.

In addition, it is also often used as an adjunct to SSRI therapy (that is, added to an SSRI) for eliminating sexual side-effects (lack of libido primarily). In general, anything that increases dopamine (particularly at the expense of serotonin or prolactin) also tends to increase sex drive.

Officially-speaking, bupropion is a *noradrenaline-dopamine reuptake inhibitor* (NDRI), with its most potent action on noradrenaline. Compared to most drugs, bupropion seems to have a wide range of opinions from researchers regarding its mechanism of action. Some believe it also works as a weak releasing agent, pumping out extra noradrenaline and dopamine. Other researchers have expressed scepticism around its dopaminergic properties, finding its clinical effects concentrated solely on noradrenaline. One thing that all seem to agree on is that its effects are relatively weak in terms of binding affinities and impact on circulating neurotransmitter levels. This is not necessarily a bad thing by the way. If it significantly jacked up dopamine, it would be associated with the rapid development of tolerance and would essentially have no point of difference compared to stimulants (and would therefore not be available as a treatment for depression).

One of the reasons why bupropion tends to feel more noradrenaline-centric than its pharmacology would suggest is due to one of its main metabolites. Hydroxybupropion, which is created when bupropion is processed in the liver by the CYP2B6 enzyme, is a strong noradrenaline reuptake inhibitor, shifting the balance away from dopamine somewhat. One of the potential manifestations of this extra noradrenaline is a side-effect you may need to watch out for – sudden, out-of-character flashes of anger. A consistent theme I have heard from those who have experienced this is for them to be suddenly overcome with anger verging on rage, triggered by something inconsequential. Sometimes it flashes up and then disappears just as quickly, leaving you thinking - What the hell was *that*? I have no reliable data on the proportion of those who experience this, however considering that I have had near identical conversations describing its features, it does give me pause for concern. Of the people who are affected, I would think that the overwhelming majority don't act on it. However if you are someone who has had anger or violence issues in the past, I would look elsewhere in terms of pharmaceuticals. Sudden, uncontrollable acts of violence have the ability to ruin lives in an instant.

One interesting thing I found when researching bupropion is that its antidepressant effects appear to be mediated by noradrenaline and less so by dopamine. When researchers give mice a drug which blocks noradrenaline, bupropion loses its antidepressant effects. However, strangely, it appears to be dopamine which gives bupropion its short term mood-boosting properties.

One of the reasons why bupropion is so effective for treating smoking cessation is because it targets two major pharmacological actions of nicotine – increased dopamine and activation of nicotinic acetylcholine (nACh) receptors. Surprisingly, bupropion does this by acting as a weak *antagonist* of nACh receptors, not agonist. This particular receptor is a little weird like that. Antagonising this receptor makes it upregulate, helping to return it to the way it functioned before it was being artificially activated by nicotine. This receptor appears to almost overshoot as it snaps back to normal, which is why nACh antagonists can help mood and act as cognitive enhancers.

Bupropion is often used for cases of depression involving a lack of motivation or energy. However for cases of anxious depression, it should be used with care as it can increase anxiety for some people. However I would consider it highly unusual if bupropion was used specifically to treat anxiety, as there is nothing in its pharmacology or real-world patient reports which would suggest efficacy or suitability. Due to its dopamine-boosting effects, social anxiety would be the only anxiety-spectrum disorder where I could imagine it being effective.

In general, one of the most useful roles which bupropion plays is as an addition to an SSRI to give an extra boost to dopamine and reduce some of the sexual side-effects usually seen with SSRIs. However in many cases (particularly where there is a lack of energy) it can be an effective monotherapy. Bupropion, like many drugs, is associated with considerable unpredictability in terms of efficacy or side-effects from person to person. Due to its fairly narrow effects, which are limited to noradrenaline and dopamine, there is really only a certain subset of cases where it would be effective. For example, compared to amitriptyline, which has a long shopping list of potent effects (both positive and negative), bupropion is highly selective and relatively weak. If you are looking for that wonder-drug to help dig yourself out of the blackest of depressive episodes or quell severe anxiety, bupropion is highly unlikely to be what you are looking for.

However, as an adjunct to a potent SSRI, bupropion can help to temper the issues which can arise from the tendency of these drugs to suppress dopamine. Most importantly, this can mitigate some of the blunted emotions and sexual dysfunction which often plague SSRIs. Unfortunately however, bupropion's usefulness as an add-on to SSRIs suffers from a major limitation. Once again, I need to return to our old friend Mr Cytochrome P450.

Whenever I thought that bupropion would be perfect for someone, due to their symptoms, at least half the time the deal breaker has been its complicated metabolism and drug interactions. First off, as mentioned a moment ago, bupropion is partially converted into hydroxybupropion by CYP2B6, which just so happens to be one of the enzymes blocked by most SSRIs. In theory, this is potentially not such a bad thing if you want more of an emphasis on dopamine instead of noradrenaline. However in practical terms, the difference is most likely insignificant. The flip-side of this is alcohol, which induces CYP2B6, so you could expect slightly more adrenergic effects.

This example is probably of most importance if bupropion was used in an alcohol detoxification process. As bupropion has anti-addictive qualities, it would not be a stretch to see it used in this context. Alcohol is often referred to as the only drug (along with benzodiazepines) where the detox process can be fatal. If you detox from heroin, you are in for a few of the most unpleasant days imaginable, however you are highly unlikely to die. However, with alcohol detox, a huge spike in adrenaline (caused by a lack of GABA and therefore a surge in glutamate) can lead to fatal seizures. This then leads on to another downside of bupropion which I will cover in a moment.

However, bupropion's complex metabolism doesn't end there. Perhaps more importantly, as well as having its own metabolism affected by CYP2B6, bupropion itself is a potent inhibitor of CYP2D6 (which is perhaps the single most important enzyme for metabolising antidepressants). This can create a hugely complex interaction between bupropion and SSRIs. For example, bupropion's conversion to hydroxybupropion is inhibited by fluoxetine and then bupropion returns the favour by inhibiting the metabolism of fluoxetine. If you are taking multiple medications, you will need to ask your doctor to check for interactions, as bupropion can affect everything from painkillers to antipsychotics to beta-blockers. If a significant interaction is identified, you will need to discuss with your doctor whether you can switch to alternative drugs not affected by bupropion, or whether bupropion will need to be avoided.

Now back to seizures, which, despite being a low probability event if bupropion is the only drug being taken, is probably the most significant risk associated with this drug. Certain drugs reduce a person's *seizure threshold*[24], and when you combine several of these, you reduce this threshold in an additive way. For example, most doctors would prescribe bupropion together with tramadol only in rare cases, as both combine to (theoretically) lower the threshold to a more significant degree compared to when each drug is taken individually.

In statistical terms, the risk of seizure with bupropion alone is still below 1% (one in a hundred chance). However as you add in other drugs which lower the threshold, this could rise to a one in twenty risk. I tend to place little faith in the overall risk numbers because, in the case of bupropion, it will be influenced by a huge number of factors such as –

- Whether you are using the extended, sustained or instant release form. When bupropion was first developed, it was banned from use because there was almost a one in twenty chance of triggering a seizure. However when they reformulated this dosage (300mg) as a sustained release tablet, the incidence dropped back below 1%
- The dosage. 300mg is more likely to cause seizures than 150mg
- Drug interactions. For example, using clomipramine with bupropion would be expected to dramatically increase the risk, however a key factor would be their CYP2D6 interaction, making things rather tricky. If you then added in tramadol, you would be heading into very dangerous territory. This is where one careless doctor can cause so much harm. For example, many people with fibromyalgia also have anxiety problems, meaning they may complain to their doctor of anxiety, pain and fatigue. So you can easily see how someone could end up with a script for bupropion, clomipramine and tramadol, if the doctor doesn't understand the interactions
- Depression itself is a risk factor for seizures. So, for example, if you combined bupropion with clomipramine, you would in one way be reducing the risk of depression-mediated seizures, but increasing the risk due to the drug interaction
- Individual genetics. Bupropion has one of the most unpredictable metabolic profiles of any drug I have encountered. At the same dose, some people can have five-times the amount of bupropion circulating in their system

Naturally, it should go without saying that if you have epilepsy, or any other seizure-related disorder, bupropion is not a good option.

The seizure issue is just something to be aware of and shouldn't cause you to completely discount bupropion as an option. At the end of the day, the risk is still quite low. I have seen many comments on internet forums where someone has been prescribed bupropion, seen reports of seizure risk and been too scared to start treatment. The irony here is that many of these people may already be taking other drugs which reduce the seizure threshold to the same degree, without knowing it.

---

[24] The threshold above which you are at risk of a seizure.

Your psychiatrist will have extensive experience in this area and will be able to put your mind at ease. If they are at all concerned regarding seizure risk (such as a history of epilepsy or seizures in your family) they will not prescribe bupropion, or they will prescribe an adjunct to bupropion to reduce any seizure risk.

Interestingly, bupropion is actually distantly related to amphetamines, however in terms of its mechanism of action (noradrenaline and dopamine reuptake inhibition), bupropion is actually more closely related to the other main stimulant used to treat ADHD – methylphenidate (Ritalin). The main difference between these two drugs is that bupropion is significantly less potent with respect to its reuptake inhibition and also has a much longer half-life. This long half-life is the reason why bupropion and methylphenidate, whilst both having approximately the same mechanism of action, are classified in completely different categories. Bupropion is an accepted, mainstream antidepressant, whereas methylphenidate is considered a stimulant and therefore is mostly used to treat ADHD.

This difference in classification is not simply a bureaucratic, arbitrary pigeonholing of these two drugs. In general, drugs with longer half-lives are preferred, as they tend to give a more stable therapeutic effect and don't require repeated dosing during the day. With bupropion, this half-life is one of main reasons why methylphenidate can be abused to "get high", whereas bupropion is widely believed to have no recreational value at all. This is why many doctors (particularly in the US) wouldn't hesitate to put someone on bupropion for depression, but would never consider using methylphenidate. There is nothing wrong with this by the way. Whilst methylphenidate can be extremely useful in certain stubborn cases of depression, it should be reserved for the exclusive prescribing benefit of specialist psychopharmacologists. In many countries this is mandated by law. For example, in Australia, any general practitioner (GP) can prescribe bupropion, however only accredited psychiatrists are allowed to prescribe methylphenidate.

To reiterate however, methylphenidate itself can be an extremely effective medication for severe, chronic or treatment resistant depression and even certain cases of social anxiety. More on methylphenidate in the section on "off-label" treatment options.

Whilst bupropion is typically available in three forms (300mg extended release, 150mg sustained release and 150mg instant release), I tend to favour the extended release forms as they don't require re-dosing later in the day (which can cause issues with insomnia) and allow for more stable blood levels.

Reboxetine *(Edronax)*

Until I created this new, updated version of the book, I had deliberately omitted reboxetine from all previous editions. For a range of reasons, I really don't like this drug, so I need to declare my unashamed negative bias on this topic. However I wondered if, by not providing information as to why I think this is a terrible drug, I might be letting slip an opportunity to guide people towards more effective medications, by outlining my case against it.

For the longest time (until 2010 to be exact), reboxetine had perplexed me. Here was a drug which every single person I spoke to said was far and away the worst antidepressant they had ever tried. This is not surprising insofar as reboxetine manages the rather impressive feat of having awful side-effects *and* being close to ineffective for depression. Its creators over at Pfizer really need to pat themselves on the back.

However, all the pieces of this puzzling jigsaw fell into place with a comprehensive and eventually, quite famous meta-analysis conducted by the *German Institute for Quality and Efficiency in Health Care* (IQWiG) and published by the *British Medical Journal* (BMJ) in 2010. When I have told this story to people, their reaction is always identical – "Pharmaceutical companies are allowed to do *what*? How is that legal?"

The reboxetine scandal is probably the single most salacious story in this book, however it is not directly linked to the topic of whether reboxetine is right for *you*, so it is a tad off-topic. I have therefore moved it to the Appendices. I strongly urge you to read the Appendix and then return to this section before you continue reading. However, considering the reason you are probably reading this book, learning about this rather scandalous state of affairs may leave you feeling worse than before, so feel free to just focus on the topic at hand.

To cut to the chase, the BMJ-published study found that -

> *"Our analysis of a comprehensive evidence base of published and unpublished trials of reboxetine compared with placebo or SSRIs in adults with major depressive disorder indicates that reboxetine is, overall, an ineffective and potentially harmful antidepressant. Published evidence on reboxetine has been substantially affected by publication bias, underlining the urgent need for mandatory publication of clinical trial data, including data on older agents."*

It would be no exaggeration to say that the above summary is the most strongly-worded conclusion of any review I have ever seen for a commonly available "antidepressant" (term used loosely).

Reboxetine is a highly-selective noradrenaline reuptake inhibitor (NRI). Think of it as methylphenidate without the "fun" or "enjoyable" part (dopamine). To be honest, I never understood the fanfare which accompanied the release of this drug. I think doctors were excited by the idea of reboxetine because –

    a) TCAs (which inhibit the reuptake of serotonin and noradrenaline) were effective but had too many side-effects caused by their lack of selectivity
    b) Reboxetine is highly selective for the noradrenaline transporter

c) Many patients don't respond to SSRIs
d) Therefore, noradrenaline may be the missing piece of the puzzle

As you may recall from earlier in the book, I often consider noradrenaline to be like salt, bringing out the natural flavours of certain food. If you add noradrenaline to dopamine, you usually get a highly pleasurable state. However an NRI (in my opinion) is like having a bowl of salt. Noradrenaline is best suited to being a spice, not a main meal. Too little and you will lack energy and motivation. Too much and you invite agitation and anxiety.

For those brave (and possibly foolhardy) souls who decide, for whatever reason, that reboxetine is just the ticket, some unpleasant side-effects await. As the BMJ review mentioned, reboxetine's side-effects are notable in their unpleasantness. For those who are able to live with the nausea, agitation, insomnia and excessive sweating (you will be quite the dinner party guest!), they will then need to ensure what is possibly the most common reason patients quite reboxetine. In my experience dealing with males who have tried reboxetine, many have reported that it became so difficult to urinate, they started to worry they would need to have a catheter put in. Due to male physiology (how the urinary tract flows through the prostate), I have not seen this issue in females (at least not to this severity). Male patients are often reduced to standing above the toilet for 10 minutes waiting for their bladder to empty, drop by drop. Fun times!

Whether it is by pure chance, or perhaps reboxetine is actually suited to a small number of people, some people report great success with it. However, based on my experience, I would guess that for every person helped, 99 aren't. Those are not odds I find particularly compelling.

Remember how I said that there is no single "best" antidepressant and that all of them are roughly the same in terms of overall efficacy? I forgot to exclude reboxetine, which is the only treatment I have ranked behind homeopathy. At least with homeopathy you get a nice drink of (99.99999% pure) water and no side-effects.

Pramipexole *(Mirapex, Sifrol)*

Pramipexole, which is primarily a treatment for restless legs and Parkinson's disease, is one of the more interesting and unusual drugs used to treat mood disorders. It is a great example of a potentially useful treatment which most doctors are unaware of[25].

---

[25] They are usually familiar with pramipexole as a treatment for RLS or Parkinson's, but not as an antidepressant

Pramipexole is a dopamine receptor agonist, which means that it activates certain dopamine receptors in the same way actual dopamine does[26]. The reason why pramipexole is interesting is that it can often work in cases where typical medications such as SSRIs have failed. This is because it works specifically on dopamine, so if your depression or anxiety is dopamine related (as opposed to serotonin or noradrenaline), you may find pramipexole worth investigation.

However there are a few caveats, as pramipexole is far from the perfect drug, despite being quite safe. Firstly, in my experience, pramipexole either works well or not at all. If I was forced to put a number on it, I would guess less than half the patients who try pramipexole actually find it useful. However if you are in the group whose problems are alleviated by pramipexole, it can be a miracle drug. I have even heard it referred to as "lifesaving" by some. If it works for you, it is a fairly strong indication that your neurochemical problems are dopaminergic in origin.

If you start taking pramipexole, bear in mind that, like SSRIs, the beginning can be unpleasant for some. I hypothesize that this is via the same mechanism seen when starting SSRIs, where the receptors initially react to the increased activation by reducing their output of neurotransmitters. This usually then normalizes within a week or so. Any drug which agonises dopamine receptors has this unfortunate aspect, where the first few days can be trying, to say the least. One thing I would recommend is to pay close attention to how you react in the first few days. If you find that the symptoms you were trying to treat become amplified, it can be a good indication that you are on the right track. When it starts to work, it should gradually begin to have the opposite effect, giving a nice boost to dopaminergic activity.

Also note that this drug has some of the weirdest (albeit rare) side effects of any drug I have seen. A small minority of patients can develop compulsive gambling and problems with hypersexuality. The out of control libido "problem" is welcomed by some. Compulsive gambling, not so much. I believe there was even a lawsuit from a patient who claimed he had gambled away his life savings after starting pramipexole.

In general, I am more comfortable with the idea of pramipexole as an antidepressant than as an anxiolytic, as dopamine is rarely the main cause of anxiety disorders (except for social anxiety). While pramipexole may be potentially useful, the start-up effects can be extremely difficult for some, giving it a fairly poor risk/return profile. One small exception is that some people find that pramipexole can help offset the sexual dysfunction caused by SSRIs, so it could have potential in some cases as an adjunct. Boosting dopamine often reduces levels of prolactin, the hormone I mentioned earlier which is released post-orgasm. Part of the cascade of

---

[26] If you are interested in learning about agonists, antagonists and everything else you need to know about neurochemistry in layman's terms, check out James Lee's well-known book on neurotransmitters and neurochemistry, *Better Living through Neurochemistry*.

effects is an increase in testosterone, which is why pramipexole is widely used in the bodybuilding/gym junkie scene for its ability to help put on muscle and reduce fat.

Mirtazapine *(Remeron, Avanza, Zispin)*

Mirtazapine is officially referred to as either a *noradrenergic and specific serotonergic antidepressant* (NaSSA) or a *tetracyclic*. Many people find mirtazapine to be an excellent sleep aid for occasional insomnia (as an alternative to benzodiazepines). Due to its mechanism of action, it can be used long term, as opposed to benzodiazepines which should usually only be used occasionally. Also, unlike benzodiazepines, mirtazapine does not impact your sleep architecture negatively, as it leaves slow-wave sleep unaffected or even increased.

However, some people believe mirtazapine should be primarily considered a sleep aid and not an anxiolytic or antidepressant. According to its marketing materials and early pharmacological studies, it exerts its effects by modulating serotonin and noradrenaline receptors, providing a mild anti-anxiety and anti-depressive effect. However by far its strongest effects are its antihistamine properties. On a "milligram for milligram" basis, mirtazapine is arguably the strongest antihistamine on the planet.

It is this antihistamine effect which is behind most of mirtazapine's side-effects and in particular, weight gain and sedation. Mirtazapine will (at least during start up), make you very sleepy and *incredibly* hungry. For some people, this sedation is a welcome development, after months (or years) of poor sleep. For others, the next-day sedation is intolerable. As a guide, if antihistamines make you feel groggy the next day, mirtazapine is probably not going to work for you. For others, it provides a wonderful, refreshing night's sleep, with increased time spent in the deepest sleep stages, providing a great restorative effect.

Mirtazapine is also miraculously free of the usual unpleasant side-effects of TCAs. In particular, it has no discernible adverse effects on the heart, a huge advantage over TCAs. If mirtazapine had been developed during the pre-SSRI era of the TCAs, it would have been viewed a miracle of modern pharmacology as it appears to have taken the best aspects of TCAs (such as improved sleep), and not the worst aspects (such as cardiotoxicity). However, crucially, mirtazapine lacks the ability to inhibit the reuptake of serotonin and noradrenaline.

This has led to a growing band of researchers who claim that mirtazapine lacks any serotonergic effects, aside from its selective antagonism of certain sub-types. Increasing serotonin levels is associated with a range of hallmarks, such as the ability to cause serotonin toxicity when combined with serotonergic drugs (particularly MAOIs) and worsened sexual function. These experts point out that not only does mirtazapine not cause serotonin syndrome, it can actually be a *treatment* for it (due to receptor antagonism). Similarly, rather than worsening sexual function, mirtazapine *improves* it, or at the very least, it is free of the sexual side-effects which plague SSRIs. In fact, it is often use as an adjunct to SSRI therapy to reduce the sexual side-effects which patients often complain of.

This points to mirtazapine's primary place in the treatment of depression and anxiety – as an additional drug to use alongside an SSRI or SNRI and not as the sole focus on pharmacological treatment. In addition to sexual side-effects, SSRIs can also worsen sleep (particularly during the start-up phase). Mirtazapine can mitigate this problem, due to its sedating and hypnotic (sleep inducing) effects.

If you find yourself intolerably sedated when starting mirtazapine, give it a little time as this quickly goes away for most people. However the weight gain and increased appetite is generally there to stay. If you are already overweight or susceptible to putting on weight, this may render mirtazapine an unrealistic option for you. However if you are severely depressed with no appetite and unhealthy weight loss, mirtazapine will be a god-send. Some people have said that mirtazapine gives you 'the munchies' just as bad as marijuana.

As mentioned previously in the section on venlafaxine, mirtazapine combined with venlafaxine, referred to as *California Rocket Fuel*, appears to be very effective as a combination therapy, so this could be worth considering. These two drugs added together appears to create a synergy which makes the combination much more effective than either drugs when used alone. At the very least, mirtazapine taken in the evening will take the edge off of any excess stimulation from the venlafaxine.

Another benefit of mirtazapine is that the withdrawal process is generally a lot milder than SSRI withdrawal. That's not to say it will be completely free of problems though. However usually the withdrawal effects are limited to transient anxiety and insomnia (as your brain gets used to sleeping without the help of mirtazapine). This is perhaps another piece of evidence against mirtazapine's debated serotonergic effects. Withdrawing from a serotonergic drug, such as an SSRI, has a distinct (and unpleasant) character which is altogether different to mirtazapine withdrawal.

One aspect of mirtazapine which I rarely see mentioned is its effects on dopamine. By antagonising the $5-HT_{2C}$ serotonin receptor, mirtazapine actually causes increased dopamine activity, as this particular receptor usually plays a role in suppressing dopaminergic neurotransmission. And importantly, it increases levels of dopamine in the reward centre of the brain, which is a pleasurable feeling that can boost mood. It is for this reason that mirtazapine is even used to treat people addicted to drugs such as methamphetamine, as it helps boost reward pathway activity, leading to reduced craving for these drugs. That said, mirtazapine's effects on dopamine are unlikely to be useful for most forms of anxiety, except perhaps for social anxiety.

Mirtazapine's ability to increase levels of dopamine is also caused by α_1-adrenergic antagonism. This is also a factor in mirtazapine's other strange property – The higher the dose, the less sedating. Most people find that, as a sleep aid, mirtazapine is more powerful at 7.5mg than 30mg. This is because as the dose increases, so too do the effects on dopamine and noradrenaline. This gradually overpowers the antihistamine effects, causing increased energy levels and improved mood. The implication of this is that for anxiety disorders, less may be more, with depression likely to benefit from higher doses (say, 30mg or so).

Although my experience with mirtazapine has been mixed, it is actually a wonder of modern drug development. For any of you who have read James Lee's *Better Living through Neurochemistry*, you would have remembered that there are a large number of receptor sub-types, such as 5-ht1a, 5-ht2c and so on. Each of these sub-types has a distinct effect when activated or blocked. This is why, as I mentioned at the start of this book, mirtazapine can be confusing for some, as they see that it blocks the activity of certain serotonin receptors. After all, aren't we trying to boost serotonergic activity? The answer is that sub receptors improve mood and reduce anxiety when activated, while others do the opposite. Mirtazapine is almost laser-like in its selectivity for doing the right thing at the right location. As an added bonus it even blocks one of the receptors involved in nausea, which is unsurprising considering its close relationship to ondansetron, a drug used primarily to treat nausea caused by morning sickness, among other things.

To summarise, mirtazapine is a fascinating drug which plays a valuable role in the treatment of anxiety and depression. While I have questions regarding just how potent it is as an antidepressant or anxiolytic, I have heard countless people report enormous benefits. Because it is one of the most powerful antihistamines in existence, it is quite possible that some or all of its effects on anxiety could be due to the sedation which antihistamines cause. Evidence of this is the fact that many people find antihistamines like promethazine and diphenhydramine to be effective anxiolytics. However I think mirtazapine's true value is as an adjunct to another drug, such as an SSRI. SSRIs indiscriminately boost serotonin all over the place, which activates certain serotonin receptors which we don't want to activate if we wish to treat anxiety. By blocking these receptors and improving sleep quality, mirtazapine can help you get the most out of your SSRI.

Also, just briefly, mirtazapine is actually the updated version of an older drug known as mianserin. If we look at their respective pharmacologies, there is nothing to really suggest any advantage for mianserin. However, it is a crazy old world out there and stranger things have happened.

Agomelatine *(Valdoxan)*

In the first edition of this book, I said the following regarding agomelatine –

> *On the plus side, this drug is relatively free from side-effects, with many psychiatrists using it when their patient has struggled with the side-effects of SSRIs. A drug which treats anxiety and depression yet with no side-effects sounds too good to be true. Especially with some of the glowing clinical trial reports which came out before it was released. Some were talking about agomelatine as a "game changer" which would cause drug companies to start focusing on melatonin receptors as the key to treating depression.*

> *However, in reality, things have been much more muted than first expectations. The vast majority of patients appear to have experienced no effects, either good or bad. Agomelatine has disparagingly been referred to be some as a "sugar pill". Another problem at the moment is cost. As it is a relatively new drug, it is still covered by patent and is therefore quite expensive, with no generic versions available yet. I have spoken to a few people who found some minor benefits taking agomelatine, however could not justify the cost with such subtle effects.*

In summary, my position on agomelatine until now has been that it is debatable whether it does anything at all, however with a low incidence of side-effects it could at least help your sleep quality improve.

However, based on more up to date research, I have now shifted my position. I would never, ever consider using agomelatine under any circumstances. Because of its lack of clinical effects, a patient risks losing 6 weeks or so, waiting for it to work, not getting better. Someone with major depression or a severe anxiety disorder should not be made to suffer needlessly, when there are so many safe and effective options.

There are also serious questions regarding its effect on the liver, with quite a bit of evidence to suggest agomelatine is toxic on the liver. It appears to be relatively common for patients taking agomelatine to have raised liver enzymes, so if you have any problems with liver function, agomelatine would be contraindicated.

Agomelatine is probably the only drug which gives reboxetine a run for its money in the "World's Most Ineffective Antidepressant" category. Therefore it probably comes as no surprise to learn that agomelatine has also been associated with the same drug company trickery as reboxetine. A review in the British Journal of Psychiatry, with the rather catchy title of *Agomelatine efficacy and acceptability revisited: systematic review and meta-analysis of published and unpublished randomised trials*, was scathing, to say the least. They obtained the results of thirteen studies, seven of which were never published by Servier, the French pharmaceutical company behind the drug. The reviewers found that none of the negative studies were ever published, so when they compare the results of published versus unpublished trials they found that there was a large discrepancy between the data, with the published trials being more positive than the unpublished trials. The review concluded –

"We found evidence suggesting that a clinically important difference between agomelatine and placebo in patients with unipolar major depression is unlikely. There was evidence of substantial publication bias."

Translation –

Agomelatine is no better than a placebo and the drug company cherry-picked which trials to publish, in order to make the drug appear effective.

After agomelatine was launched with much fanfare in 2005, gradually word spread between doctors and patients that agomelatine simply didn't work. At all. Then things went from bad to worse with a flurry of bad press after a prominent (and otherwise well-respected) Australian psychiatrist, Professor Ian Hickie, published a paper in The Lancet which spoke of agomelatine in glowing terms. This triggered immense criticism of Professor Hickie due to a range of factors, however the primary reason was that his paper was clearly at odds with the body of evidence available on agomelatine's efficacy. This story is compelling reading, as it manages to serve as a perfect example of what is wrong with the pharmaceutical industry. However, rather than stray too far from the purpose of this book, I have included a summary in the appendices which was published in an Australian publication for GPs and other doctors.

One thing I will acknowledge is that I like the fact that a drug company tried to treat depression from a different angle, rather than just putting out another "me too" SSRI. For what it's worth, agomelatine is a *melatonin receptor agonist*, theoretically activating the receptors for the hormone you usually produce to control your circadian rhythm (body clock). If disrupted sleep cycles are behind your issues, this could be helpful. Theoretically, it is supposed to also act as a weak serotonin receptor antagonist, which may (or may not) contribute to any benefits with mood or anxiety, via a similar mechanism as mirtazapine. Just like mirtazapine, agomelatine is extremely selective. It acts as an antagonist at the 5-HT_{2C} receptor, which would usually result in increased levels of dopamine and noradrenaline.

Agomelatine is one of those drugs which looks awesome on paper, yet this doesn't translate to real-world clinical effects. A drug which is able to improve sleep quality by normalising your circadian rhythm (which tends to be disrupted in people with mood disorders), as well as boosting dopamine and noradrenaline would be a smash hit. However agomelatine has been anything but. In its short and chequered history, agomelatine has been knocked back by various health agencies such as the European Medicines Agency, who weren't satisfied with its efficacy[27].

However the most striking example of agomelatine's lack of efficacy was when North American marketing rights were assigned to Novartis, who planned on then submitting an application to the FDA after the completion of Phase III trials. When

---

[27] They somehow re-applied the following year and were granted approval, with certain restrictions.

Novartis saw the results of these trials, they didn't even bother going through with the application to the FDA. This is why it is not available in the US.

Despite everything I have just said about agomelatine, you may be shocked to learn that I know a few people who are taking it and they love it! One even said that the effects were so potent, agomelatine felt almost "recreational". Agomelatine is also one of the few drugs in this book that I have direct experience with. A few years ago I was doing a lot of international travel, at one stage going on four round-the-world trips in two years. I felt like my body clock was shot so I thought I would give agomelatine a go for its effects on melatonin.

It did absolutely nothing. At all.

Vortioxetine *(Brintellix)*

Vortioxetine is the "new kid on the block" in the antidepressant market, receiving approval from the FDA (for major depression) in 2013. While it is probably a little too early to say with confidence that it will be as effective as SSRIs, I was pleased to see it get released. The pipeline of new antidepressants has dried up in recent years, with drug companies switching their focus to more profitable niches such as statins.

To a certain extent, antidepressants have become a victim of their own success. Because we have a large selection of effective SSRIs and SNRIs (not to mention the older TCAs and MAOIs), to gain approval in Europe and North America, any new drug must demonstrate, at the very least, efficacy approximating the existing drugs. Many don't even make it past initial trials and many are rejected by the FDA, while others scrape through and get released, only to bomb badly with patients and doctors.

I also like the fact that vortioxetine has a mechanism of action which is quite distinct, officially referred to as a *serotonin modulator and stimulator*, due to its unusual combination of effects. Vortioxetine's pharmacodynamics which contribute to its putative antidepressant effects are –

- It is a fairly potent SSRI
- It is a weak noradrenaline reuptake inhibitor
- It is a serotonin receptor agonist at certain receptors
- It is a serotonin antagonist at other receptors

If the efficacy of antidepressants could be easily predicted by looking at their binding affinities and *in-vitro* effects, vortioxetine would be a blockbuster. It's not often I look at the pharmacology of a drug and think *wow – that is impressive*. If you were to work through each serotonin sub-receptor, from $5-HT_{1A}$ through to $5-HT_7$, choosing which ones to antagonise and which ones to agonise, vortioxetine does all the right things at all the right receptors. Also, don't forget that, similar to mirtazapine, antagonising certain serotonin receptors leads to increased levels of dopamine and noradrenaline in certain parts of the brain. Interestingly, whereas mirtazapine does this via the 5-HT$_{2c}$ receptor, vortioxetine acts via 5-HT$_3$. This also means that each drug boosts dopamine and noradrenaline in different parts of the brain. However, generally speaking, vortioxetine appears to be significantly more potent in this regard.

This highlights a point I have touched on previously. When I say *"boosts dopamine levels"*, I am making a gross simplification in the interests of keeping this book readable. For this statement to be of any use, a neuroscientist would need to know *where* exactly dopamine levels are increasing. In this regard, vortioxetine easily has the most complicated effects on serotonin, dopamine and noradrenaline of any drug I have seen. It specifically boosts these neurotransmitters in some places but not others. For example, it boosts dopamine and noradrenaline in places like the prefrontal cortex, but not the nucleus accumbens. Boosting these two neurotransmitters in your reward centres (including the nucleus accumbens) is associated with addictive drugs like cocaine. Despite the fact that this would be pleasurable, in general this is not a desired effect when you are treating depression, as activating this pathway tends to only work the first few times you take the drug in question, before tolerance sets in.

Because vortioxetine boosts dopamine and noradrenaline in the prefrontal cortex, it has pro-cognitive effects, potentially normalising some of the cognitive dysfunction (poor concentration, clouded thinking etc.) seen in cases of major depression. This effect is further boosted by vortioxetine's ability to increase levels of acetylcholine and histamine, an interesting property considering antidepressants have always tended to be the complete opposite – anticholinergic and antihistaminergic.

Due to its pharmacology and general feedback from patients, vortioxetine has limited use in the treatment of anxiety disorders, as it can be a rather anxiogenic drug. This may be accentuated by the effects on acetylcholine and histamine.

Vortioxetine's single greatest drawback is its effects on gastrointestinal function and in particular, nausea. Some people assume that this is due to its effects on serotonin (with SSRIs and diarrhoea being well known), however it is more likely that dopamine is the culprit, due to dopamine's central role in modulating the process underlying nausea. Whilst nausea appears to be the most common side-effect, others just report continual GI distress.

As I always say – there is no such thing as a free lunch. With increased potency usually comes increased side-effects. While this may be a price someone with severe depression is willing to pay, for mild to moderate cases, there just isn't enough compelling evidence to say that vortioxetine could be an effective first line treatment. Coupled with this is the fact that it is a new drug which is still patent protected and is therefore quite expensive. In some countries with universal healthcare or for people with good insurance coverage, this is not such an issue. However for those on a tight budget, with such a huge number of different (cheaper) options, the rationale for selecting vortioxetine as the first drug you go on, is weak.

Being a new drug also means that there are not enough real-world cases with which we can form a reliable view on efficacy. When I researched this drug, the vast majority of comments online were negative, however it is unclear how much weight should be given to these comments when forming your own view.

Vilazodone *(Viibryd)*

First of all, am I the only one who thinks that "vilazodone" and "Viibryd" are terrible names for an antidepressant? I assume that "Viibryd" is designed to convey the word vibrant, however I don't think it works. And when I read "vilazodone", I just see the word "vile" or "evil".

That reminds me, you may have heard the interesting background to how certain drugs are named and even the colour of the pills. "Relaxing" drugs like benzodiazepines usually have blue pills as this is supposed to convey some kind of extra efficacy. Just goes to show that even drugs with active ingredients also do everything they can to harness the placebo effect like homeopathy does. I first heard about this when I saw a study which showed that branded OTC paracetamol (acetaminophen) like Tylenol or Panadol had a stronger painkilling effect because the people taking them associated the branded version with potency or efficacy. We humans certainly can be weird sometimes.

Anyhoo…you may file the above two paragraphs away in a drawer marked "useless". I thought after making it this far into a book on antidepressants, you deserved a two-paragraph time-out.

Vilazodone is another recently developed drug, gaining approval from the FDA for the treatment of major depression in 2011. Like vortioxetine, vilazodone attempts to build on SSRIs by adding in serotonin receptor agonism, in the hope that this addresses some of the shortcomings of existing drugs. Vilazodone has even been placed in the rather fancy-named category *serotonin partial agonist reuptake inhibitor* (SPARI), which is kind of pointless at this stage as vilazodone is currently the sole member of this particular club.

As the name suggests, vilazodone's sole differentiating factor is the partial agonism of 5-ht$_{1a}$, in addition to its SSRI properties. Whether vilazodone ends up being more effective (or even *as* effective) as SSRIs, remains to be seen. However I have to give the developers kudos for trying, as 5-ht$_{1a}$ agonism has long been touted as a way to mitigate some of the deficiencies of SSRIs.

For reasons which are long, complicated and ultimately, rather boring[28], it is believed that the 5-ht$_{1a}$ receptor is a key player in the therapeutic lag which is a huge issue with antidepressant therapy. Whereas some people can take up to 12 weeks before they reach peak therapeutic effects, vilazodone is reported to be able to reduce this down to a more respectable 2 weeks.

5-ht$_{1a}$ receptor (partial) agonism is also the reason for vilazodone's theoretical (or at best, putative) ability to reduce the sexual dysfunction associated with SSRIs. Like just about everything with new drugs like these, almost everything is theoretical. We just don't have a large enough sample size from the general population which would give me confidence in vouching for the potential benefits of vilazodone. To use sexual dysfunction as an example, the best we can do is say –

1. Drugs that act as 5-ht$_{1a}$ receptor agonists tend to reduce the sexual dysfunction associated with SSRIs;
2. The drug buspirone is also a 5-ht$_{1a}$ receptor (partial) agonist and it is often effective as reducing sexual dysfunction in patients taking SSRIs
3. Vilazodone is an SSRI + 5-ht$_{1a}$ receptor (partial agonist)
4. Therefore, vilazodone *may* be associated with less sexual dysfunction compared to straight SSRIs

Interestingly, the use of buspirone together with SSRIs for increased anxiolytic effect and reduced sexual dysfunction highlights a very useful property of vilazodone, if it eventually proves as effective as the rodent trials and binding assays showed. When you are first started on an SSRI, typically the doctor will want you to go through the start-up phase until you are either stable or it becomes clear that a different drug is warranted. Most will avoid the addition of buspirone from the start as it will not be clear which drug is doing what. If you end up not responding to one or even two SSRIs, it will be months before buspirone can be added (and you will then need to wait for buspirone to take effect). Vilazodone holds the promise of being able to achieve this right at the start, and if it ends up working as desired, you have potentially avoided months of unpleasantness.

For newer drugs like vilazodone, things become a bit "chicken and egg". We want more real-world user reports or trial data before doctors and patients feel sufficiently comfortable that the drug is safe and effective. However, at least at the start, this can be the very thing that impedes this data from being generated. The first wave of patients therefore tend to be those who are long-term, sporadic users of antidepressants who have become treatment-resistant. Each new drug such as vilazodone tends to hold promise for these people (of whom you may be one) who may wonder hopefully, *maybe this will finally be the one*. Until then, all we have are

---

[28] For those interested, the 5-ht1a receptor controls the initial response to an SSRI, where everything quickly downregulates in the presence of extra serotonin, before gradually normalising over a period of weeks.

rodent trials, pre-release clinical trials (in which you may place varying degrees of confidence…*reboxetine anyone?*) and impressive test-tube level properties. So unless you are a rat or a mouse (and if so, why are you reading this? Or, for that matter, *how* are you reading this?) you may want to exhaust other, more proven options while waiting for more evidence to accumulate.

Tianeptine *(Stablon)*

Tianeptine is possibly the most underrated and underused antidepressant I know of. It is yet another European drug which somehow never received approval for major depression in the USA. In fact, it appears as if the French patent holders (Servier) never bothered to apply to the FDA, due perhaps to cost versus the probability of it receiving approval. Again we have the suspiciously inexplicable situation where another European drug is unavailable for American patients. Tianeptine is potentially a victim of its own success, demonstrating a huge number of beneficial effects which includes one or two which attract unwanted attention from regulators. I will explain why in a minute.

The existence and effectiveness of tianeptine is a headache for those who believe that the "only" way to treat depression is by inhibiting the reuptake of serotonin with SSRIs. This is because tianeptine is a *selective serotonin re-uptake enhancer*. Yes, you read that correctly. In terms of its serotonergic activity, it works in the exact opposite way to SSRIs, yet acts as an effective antidepressant.

I see tianeptine as the perfect example of my oft-repeated mantra – There is no single disorder called "depression" or "anxiety", as these are simply labels used to represent a constellation of symptoms. Both you and your best friend may have been diagnosed with major depression or generalised anxiety, however your symptoms may seem quite different. You may be lethargic, finding it difficult to even get out of bed, while your friend may be constantly agitated, unable to sleep. A good psychiatrist will be able to distil all of these symptoms down to a particular drug. Failing that, by the end of this book, you will be able to get closer than most primary care doctors (GPs) can in working out the most logical starting place.

Based on its pharmacology, I think tianeptine works as an antidepressant for reasons not directly related to serotonin re-uptake. Or say for a minute that you have the choice of tianeptine or and SSRI and you (or your doctor) must decide on one or the other as the most likely to work. And then let's assume you then visit another doctor for a second opinion. Depending on the doctor and their familiarity with tianeptine, you could literally walk out of each office with a prescription for drugs which have the opposite effect to one another!

So how come tianeptine is such an effective drug, yet appears to reduce levels of serotonin instead of increasing levels, as the SSRIs do?

One of the most plausible explanations is that by suppressing serotonin, tianeptine boosts levels of dopamine and noradrenaline. My real world experience tallies with this. Most patients I talk to report that it *feels* dopaminergic. In addition, another useful aspect of tianeptine is that it also acts as weak opioid agonist, an action shared with opiate painkillers, albeit at significantly less potent levels. As opiates themselves can act as short term powerful antidepressants and anxiolytics, this should not be surprising. This (frankly, fairly insignificant) opioid activity is what complicates things when health regulators conduct their assessments. In some parts of the world, any mention of the word "opioid" triggers a big red panic button, leading some of the more "scientifically-challenged" countries to recognise it as an illegal drug of abuse.

Surprisingly, tianeptine is technically (at least chemically) a TCA, yet somehow manages to avoid all of the deficiencies which afflict TCAs as a class, such as cardiotoxicity and anticholinergic side-effects. In fact, compared to most antidepressants, the side-effect profile is pretty good, with headaches and dizziness the main issues you may need to watch out for.

I think perhaps the most salient aspect of tianeptine's complex pharmacology is its effects on glutamate, modulating NMDA and AMPA activity. Later in the book (in the Off-label section), I will explain what NMDA and AMPA are and why the glutamatergic system is increasingly the subject of research focus.

Not convinced? What if I told you, in addition to the above, tianeptine -

- Turbo-charges neuroplasticity by ramping up levels of BDNF. Considering that depression is associated with atrophy of the hippocampus, and tianeptine literally acts as fertiliser for the regrowth process, you can see how beneficial it can be
- Possesses an additional neuroplastic action which is relatively unique. Tianeptine appears to prevent the negative adaptations of the amygdala during chronic stress. An amygdala which has gone haywire is a central feature of both depression and anxiety disorders
- Prevents the cascade of negative effects in the brain which usually occur during a period of chronic stress (which itself is one of the most common triggers for depression
- Blocks the ability of pro-inflammatory cytokines to damage the brain during stressful experiences. Again, as neural inflammation is implicated in major depression, this has huge potential as a neuroprotective agent.
- Trials have consistently demonstrated that tianeptine is at least as effective as SSRIs and potentially more so
- In contrast to many drugs (in particular, TCAs), tianeptine actually improves cognitive performance, which is why it is popular in the nootropics community.

Tianeptine appears to be particularly effective for anxiety, so it could be one of your first options if SSRIs don't work and you have either straight anxiety or anxious depression. However, as with anything that boosts dopamine, I suspect it is better for social anxiety than other types. Tianeptine also appears to be comparatively free of the side-effects usually associated with SSRIs, making it a potentially useful option if you are unable to tolerate SSRI-related side-effects.

I have generally found tianeptine to be one of those drugs which doesn't work for everyone, however when it does work, it *really, really* works. Some patients are astounded at how it can completely obliterate anxiety and depression. To be honest, tianeptine is one of those drugs which probably should be more widely used as a second-line treatment, however most doctors are either completely unaware of its existence or they don't have sufficient experience or confidence in prescribing. It isn't even available to buy at all in Australia, for example. I suspect that some of the reluctance to prescribe tianeptine comes from the fact that it has mild opioid activity, which can spook some doctors who may be concerned about addictiveness or coming under scrutiny for prescribing such a medication for depression. There are probably also many primary care doctors (GPs) who are scared off by the fact that tianeptine enhances the reuptake of serotonin, not fully understanding the complete pharmacological picture. One of the most common problems I see is the *doctor-effect*, where patients always assume that the doctor knows everything. In my experience, most GPs have only the most rudimentary understanding of neurochemistry and pharmacology, as they must be a *jack of all trades*, knowing just enough to be able to prescribe something or on-send you to a psychiatrist.

Tianeptine is one of those medications which sits at the crossroads of a range of applications. It has become fairly popular in nootropic circles, with many users reporting improved cognitive abilities. Unsurprisingly, it is classified differently in different countries. This is the reason why a sizable minority of users buy it via the internet, where it is available on various sites. If you are determined to try it, then this may be an option for you, depending on your country's import regulations. Most people report having no issues in terms of customs seizures. However, to reiterate a regular theme in this guide, in general your best strategy is to work with a clinical psychiatrist, who will either be able to prescribe tianeptine or will be able to identify an alternative option.

Trazodone *(Desyrel)*

Trazodone is a fairly unique drug, belonging to the rather sparse *serotonin receptor antagonist and re-uptake inhibitor* (SARI) class, with perhaps vilazodone (or, at a stretch, buspirone) as its closest relative amongst the drugs covered in this book. It acts as an antagonist for all serotonin receptor sub-types except for 5-HT$_{1A}$, where it acts as a partial agonist, similar to buspirone. Despite its official status as a reuptake inhibitor, its effect on the SERT transporter is so weak it can almost be disregarded. In fact, trazodone's effects on various receptors and transporters are incredibly complex because there are dramatic differences in potency for each. This also means that the effects of trazodone can change markedly depending on the dose, because as the dose increases, some of these activities cross the minimum threshold required to be clinically noticeable.

In addition to the above, trazodone also blocks the α_1-adrenergic receptor like mirtazapine, sometimes leading to side-effects such as orthostatic hypotension (where you become dizzy when you stand up from being seated for a while).

Trazodone's pharmacologic activity is further complicated by one of its metabolites - *meta-chlorophenylpiperazine* (mCPP). When your body metabolises trazodone, it essentially creates this entirely new drug. The problem with mCPP is that it has almost the exact opposite properties than trazodone itself. Or, put another way, if you were to simply take mCPP as a drug, it would worsen depression and make you even more anxious. So I think that one of the main factors which determines whether trazodone is effective for you is how your liver processes it. Trazodone is metabolised by CYP3A4, so if we take into account the wide genetic variation in everyone's cytochrome P450 activity, your response to trazodone could be heavily influence by this. I can't help but feel that trazodone's usefulness is hampered by this unfortunate property.

Trazodone is most effective for anxiety disorders, however can also be useful in treating depression. This is partially due to the sedating effect. Trazodone is an excellent sleep aid for this reason. I would hazard a guess that in the US, trazodone is used more as a sleep aid than as an anxiolytic. As it is not available in some countries, doctors will often use mirtazapine instead if the situation calls for anxiolysis or sedation.

While trazodone has a relatively mild side-effect profile, it can be associated with anticholinergic effects like dry mouth, blurred vision and dizziness. There are also several more serious, albeit rarer side-effects to all bear in mind. Like TCAs, trazodone can also have an impact on heart rhythms. Also, it can be occasionally associated with priapism, where a male experiences an erection that will not go down. There have also been rare reports of negative effects on the liver – however these are sufficiently rare that they do not usually impact the decision to try trazodone.

Aripiprazole *(Abilify)*

As you have seen, there are a range of augmentation strategies which can be used to either increase the efficacy of an antidepressant or to mitigate some of the side-effects. One such augmentation strategy is the addition of the atypical antipsychotic *aripiprazole* to an SSRI to achieve better rates of response.

In general, if you hear the word "antipsychotic" mentioned outside the context of disorders such as schizophrenia or schizoaffective disorder (such as the use of Seroquel/quetiapine as a sleep aid for insomniacs), you should promptly turn around and make for the nearest exit. While the newer atypical antipsychotics (not to be confused with atypical *antidepressants*) such as quetiapine are a significant improvement over the older, first generation drugs, this class tends to be serious, powerful stuff, with a range of side-effects which, whilst being a price that schizophrenic patients would gladly pay, rarely has justification in relatively more straightforward mood disorders.

However aripiprazole has a novel pharmacological profile which lends itself to the occasional use in augmentation strategies where the antidepressant alone is not sufficient.

In terms of its ability to treat anxiety and depression, aripiprazole appears to work as a partial agonist of D_2 (and to a lesser extent, D_3 and D_4) dopamine receptors. This is where aripiprazole differs from the other drugs typical of this class. Generally-speaking, the treatment of schizophrenic type disorders is based around dopamine antagonists. Abnormally high dopaminergic activity is behind most examples of psychosis, whether it be due to an underlying disorder such as schizophrenia or the amphetamine psychosis seen in hard-core methamphetamine addicts. So whilst dopamine antagonists are great at ameliorating psychotic symptoms, by blocking dopaminergic function, they can also block a person's ability to feel pleasure. This is clearly not an ideal outcome for someone wishing to treat depression. However aripiprazole circumvents this shortcoming, opening up its occasional use in mood disorders.

In addition to its dopamine (partial) agonist effects, aripiprazole also functions as a mixed serotonin agonist/antagonist (depending on the receptor sub-type). Interestingly, as certain receptors, aripiprazole has virtually the opposite effect to mirtazapine. This is interesting for two reasons.

Firstly, it highlights that aripiprazole should rarely be a first-line option, combined with an SSRI from day one of treatment, as it has some actions which are in direct contrast to those typically associated with improved mood or reduced anxiety. Or, put another way, if a psychiatrist wanted to augment from day one, in the absence of any psychotic symptoms, rarely would they sequence aripiprazole ahead of mirtazapine.

Secondly, if we stick with mirtazapine, one of the factors which makes that drug a kind of "weight gain perfect storm" is its 5-ht_{2c} antagonism (in addition to its antihistamine effects, which are usually considered to be the primary factor). This particular receptor is a key factor in appetite and weight control. However aripiprazole has the opposite effect, meaning it is also less associated with the often astounding weight gain seen with the other antipsychotics. This doesn't mean that you won't gain weight – you almost certainly will (and probably more than you would see with antidepressants including SSRIs and even mirtazapine), however not to the level of other drugs in this class.

However, in general, due to the extra side-effects it can cause when added to an SSRI, aripiprazole is generally only used for *treatment-resistant depression* that hasn't responded to SSRIs. Its dopaminergic activity means that it can be associated with some fairly serious (yet, I should add, extremely rare) side-effects such as *neuroleptic malignant syndrome* and *tardive dyskinesia*.

While most antidepressants are also effective anxiolytics, there are a range of drugs aimed fairly and squarely at anxiety only. So in general (with one or two exceptions), the drugs in this category possess no antidepressant characteristics as such. However, these drugs can have a beneficial effect on mood due to the relief of anxiety. As any anxiety sufferer knows, any drug which acutely reduces anxiety will put you in a good mood.

As I have written elsewhere, sometimes your mood is dictated by how your brain perceives this moment, compared to the moment which preceded it. If I told you right now that you don't have to go to jail, it would probably have no effect on your mood. However if you were sitting in the docks, awaiting the jury's decision in a case where you are accused of murder, and you heard the words *not guilty*, you would probably be ecstatic. This would be because, in the moment prior, you were suffering, as you envisaged the death penalty or life imprisonment. In this example, hearing you will not go to jail has a *much* different flavour.

What I have tried to convey via the above (frankly, rather clunky and ham-fisted) analogy is that specifically targeting anxiety, when you have either an anxiety disorder or anxious depression, can be an effective means to improve mood also. A chronic pain sufferer who takes a drug which relieves their pain experiences the same phenomenon. Chronic pain unfortunately goes hand in hand with depression, as anyone who has injured their back could probably imagine. However sometimes, just treating the pain is enough.

However it should also be noted that for some, anxiolytics such as the benzodiazepine class, can, over time, worsen mood due to their suppression of energy levels. Sometimes this is simply a matter of giving dosages a tune, so that you are able to strike the right balance between eliminating anxiety and lethargy.

The main distinction between the drugs in this category and the previous categories is that they are pharmacologically distinct. Whereas serotonin, dopamine and noradrenaline hold primacy in the antidepressant category, in this section, much of the pharmacological activity is centred on GABA and glutamate. The drugs in this section typically work independent of serotonin, dopamine or noradrenaline, aside from knock-on effects when mood improves.

For anxious depression, your doctor will almost always go with an antidepressant that works via serotonin, as it will target both anxiety and mood concurrently. Alternatively, for more severe cases, a dedicated anxiolytic may be added to the antidepressant. Similarly, many specialists like to use an anxiolytic as a short term option for dealing with the anxiety which can manifest when starting an SSRI.

Benzodiazepines (often referred to as *benzos*) are the spectacularly effective, yet imperfect "gold standard" cornerstone of the treatment of severe anxiety disorders, the management of anxiety disorders which have not responded to SSRIs and indeed for managing the initial anxiety caused by SSRIs when first started. In contrast to many other medications, benzodiazepines can give relief from anxiety in around thirty minutes. This compares to SSRIs, which take around three weeks to start providing any relief from anxiety. This makes them invaluable in emergency situations like panic attacks or where someone with a severe phobia is required to expose themselves to whatever it is they fear (such as taking a plane flight).

All benzodiazepines work by enhancing the action of gamma amino butyric acid (GABA) in your brain, which as I mentioned earlier, is the primary "calming" or *inhibitory* neurotransmitter in your brain, putting the brake on mental activity, including anxiety. Of all the drugs in this book, benzos are perhaps the most difficult to convey in terms of their mechanism of action. They are enigmatic in this sense because as long as you talk in general terms, sticking to *"they increase the activation of the GABA$_A$ receptors, thereby calming neuronal excitability"*, everything looks quite simple and at this level, they look almost simplistic compared to the more complex drugs like amitriptyline. After all – one neurotransmitter, one receptor sub-type.

Whereas an SSRI works by ensuring that there is much more serotonin floating around, benzos don't boost the amount of GABA per se, they just increase the activation of GABA$_A$ receptors. This is where things get rather complicated and probably unnecessary for me to get too tied up in for the purposes of this book (to which you possibly exclaimed - *That hasn't stopped you before!*). The best way to explain it is that the GABA$_A$ receptor, while being a sub-type of the GABA receptor itself, also has a (frankly, confusing) number of further sub-types, usually involving obscure Greek letters of the alphabet such as (α, β and γ). Imagine the GABA$_A$ receptor, which is activated by GABA itself, and then imagine these sub-types in the gaps between two GABA$_A$ receptors. Some of these are the ones activated by benzos. Perhaps unsurprisingly, these have been named the benzodiazepine receptors (BzR).

There are countless types of benzos, however only a handful of these are actually available to use. While each benzo shares the same common mechanism, there is actually surprising diversity between them. In general, temazepam is the only one used as a sleeping tablet per se, with the rest reserved for anxiety of various description. The main difference between each benzo is the pharmacokinetic profile, with certain drugs taking longer to start working and then remain active for longer.

However, there are many downsides. Firstly, they *can* be addictive for some people, so this needs to be monitored carefully. Most psychiatrists prefer not to use benzos for long term treatment, except in the most severe cases of anxiety or panic disorder. They also impact your sleep architecture, robbing you of valuable deep (*slow wave*) sleep. In the case of short term use this is fine, but longer term this is not ideal, as your brain that needs all the deep sleep it can get, as this is the stage of sleep where neurotransmitters are replenished.

In contrast to SSRIs, benzodiazepines are considered neurotoxic, whereas SSRIs are generally neurotrophic. The word neurotoxic can sometimes create alarm, however it is important to point out that at the doses the average anxiety-sufferer takes benzos, any effects are likely to be either mild or non-existent. Benzos are a (sometimes vital) Band-Aid. While you are taking them, they are not repairing or rewiring your brain, like the neurotrophic effects we see with SSRIs and their effects on the amygdala and hippocampus.

In effect this means that it is important you stick to the minimum effective dose and never take more than is prescribed to you. The results of long term, high-dose benzo abuse are not pretty. If you want to see this first-hand as way of maintaining willpower while taking a benzo, look up video from one of those (admittedly awful, for a range of reasons) television programs such as *Intervention* or *Addicted*.

If it turns out that you require indefinite treatment with a benzo, you will probably need to accept that there will be some cognitive and psycho-motor effects. You are essentially treating anxiety by turning the dimmer switch down in your brain, which means that anxiety decreases, but so too does brain function. MRI scans clearly show that they reduce activity in important parts of the brain such as the pre-frontal cortex and can impair memory. However as long as they are not abused, these effects should be either minor or imperceptible.

One of the most important things to bear in mind with benzodiazepines is that, along with alcohol, they are extremely dangerous to withdraw from if you have been on a high dose for a long time. Among all the various drugs (including drugs of abuse like heroin and cocaine), benzodiazepines and alcohol are the only two that carry risk of death if done too quickly or without proper medical supervision. If you have been on benzo therapy for a while or at a high dose, never stop taking your medication suddenly or even tapering down of your own volition without the supervision of your doctor. I spend quite a bit of time following internet forums to get a sense of peoples' experiences with certain drugs. Many times I have read about heroin addicts or people abusing other "hard" drugs referring quite flippantly to heroin withdrawal. Yet when the topic turns to benzos, these same people can refer to benzo withdrawal in grave, ominous tones, saying that heroin withdrawal is a "walk in the park" by comparison. If you stop heroin cold turkey, you are in for a few excruciating days, however if you were to do the same with a high dose benzo dependence and you could quite literally die. People are often surprised to hear that among all the various nasty drugs out there, a commonly prescribed sleeping tablet and alcohol (at alcoholic-level doses) are the only ones that can kill you if you are not careful.

Also, while I am on the topic of alcohol, please note that benzos should never, ever be combined with alcohol. Combining these two (especially in larger amounts), carries a very real risk of death. You have probably heard of famous cases where an actor or a singer has overdosed with a benzo in their system. Whilst you are unlikely to perish after having a glass of wine with your medication, it's not worth the risk as there are just too many factors which influence your reaction.

While it is *theoretically* possible to overdose by taking a large dose of benzos (however unlikely), most problems are the result of the combination of benzos and alcohol or an opiate of some kind. The main danger with *downer* combinations is that they have an additive effect which can slow down your breathing to a much greater extent than each downer alone.

I wanted to clearly outline the drawbacks of benzos, as sometimes I talk to people who have expressed frustration at their doctor's unwillingness to prescribed benzos. While I think that sometimes this unfortunately results on severe anxiety going undertreated, with a doctor dogmatically clinging to the notion that benzos are to be avoided, most of the time this is probably the right call. Benzos are typically best left for short-term use (such as during SSRI start-up or during a time-limited, atypical period of anxiousness), occasional emergency use (for phobic and panic disorders) or for when everything has been tried, yet with limited success.

However I am not going to join in the chorus of hysterical people saying that *"Xanax should be banned"* or something equally off the mark. The overwhelming majority of people who use this class of drugs do so responsibly. For people with severe anxiety and panic, benzodiazepines can restore quality of life, which should be the overriding goal. If any of these people had to endure a single day of what someone with severe anxiety has to learn to deal with, I think they would agree. It is incredibly rare for a benzo to not reduce anxiety dramatically, so it would be illogical to forgo certain benefits due to a small chance of addiction or future cognitive problems. I would contend that untreated anxiety and depression can often be much more damaging on the brain. Even just chronically elevated cortisol is more damaging than sensible treatment of anxiety with a benzo.

These days, benzodiazepine drugs are being prescribed less and less, due to better options being available in most cases. Before the existence of SSRIs, benzos were a necessary tool for the treatment of anxiety, however now, those in the moderate category for severity can usually be managed with escitalopram or one of the other SSRIs. Even severe anxiety will usually respond to a more potent option such as paroxetine. However for severe panic disorder or debilitating forms of generalised anxiety disorder, benzos remain the most effective treatment in many cases.

They are also effective sleep aids for short term use, with many doctors still prescribing temazepam when a patient complains of insomnia. To be honest, I find this perplexing, because these days there are alternative sleep aids which don't impact sleep quality like benzos do. Depending on the person, doctors should usually try to stick to other options like zolpidem, zopiclone, mirtazapine or even pregabalin. However many doctors remain stuck in their ways and haven't adapted as new agents become available, still mindlessly writing out scripts for temazepam despite the availability of better options.

As mentioned previously, one of the most important uses for this class of drugs is for short-term use when a patient starts SSRI therapy for depression or anxiety. Due to the fact that starting an SSRI is often associated with increased anxiety, benzodiazepine drugs can be extremely helpful in making the first week or two bearable, enabling the patient to see out the therapy. However, once the initial period is over and the patient has stabilised on the SSRI, benzodiazepines should be gradually withdrawn to avoid the development of physical dependency. Another important point is that these drugs can sometimes actually *worsen* depression, so should always be used only briefly or in small doses if you are also suffering from depression. Particularly for lethargic depression, it is going to be difficult to regain your energy levels if you remain perpetually under the influence of sedating drugs like benzos.

To reiterate, please don't take all of my cautionary explanations to mean that you shouldn't consider this class of drug. The problems I describe are mostly a consequence of reckless abuse, dangerous combinations and cold turkey detox. If you are prescribed a benzodiazepine indefinitely and you stick to a sensible dose and don't abuse them, they are relatively safe to take long term and can be a god-send when all else fails.

If you have severe, disabling, and intractable anxiety (particularly panic disorder, agoraphobia or in rare cases, OCD), and both you and your doctor have decided that a benzo is required, after a week or so, you will almost certainly view it as a miracle drug. There are literally millions of people around the world who have been given their life back by a benzo. In terms of the net effect across all patients, benzos would come close to being the drug that has alleviated more mental suffering than any other. You just need to go into the process with eyes wide open. No one should ever leave a doctor's office with a script for a benzo without receiving detailed information regarding the risks and various cautionary aspects of this class.

There are two types of anxiety disorder which don't really respond as well to a benzo – OCD and PTSD. This is possibly because OCD tends to primarily be a serotonin-related disorder. While a benzo is going to reduce the anxiety component of OCD, they don't tend to treat the obsessional aspect. Similarly, PTSD involves a fairly distinct neural process which is more closely linked with noradrenaline than GABA.

A recurring theme you may have noticed in this book is a strategy whereby your deeper understanding of the different medications as a whole, along with the different actions of each drug, enables you to arrive at a regime involving a lower number of individual drugs. Co-morbidity of conditions is incredibly common when there is a mood disorder present. For example, as mentioned elsewhere, the average fibromyalgia patient is on six different drugs. In general, the fewer medications you can get by on, the better. Each additional medication brings with it various side-effects and interactions with existing drug. For example, a common one I see a lot is where someone is taking opiate-based pain medication and then they start taking an SSRI, only to find the pain medication stops working. As I have shown with your P450 liver enzymes, not only do individuals have differing levels of P450 activity, depending on the drugs involved, they can either make each other less powerful or more powerful. So if you are taking morphine or oxycodone and you then start an SSRI, you will potentially lose a small amount of effectiveness due to SSRIs' anti-dopaminergic properties. However, if you are taking codeine, there is the chance that it will almost completely stop working, as codeine requires conversion to morphine in the liver, using P450 enzymes, and most SSRIs block certain subtypes such as CYP2D6 etc. However if your drug regime is uncomplicated, there is less need to worry about the various minor interactions (however you still need to take into consideration the "big" ones like MAOIs).

In some cases however, the addition of another drug is actually beneficial to the existing drug, through *potentiation*. This is fantastic when we are talking about drugs whose side-effect profile jumps as the dose escalates. For example, many fibromyalgia sufferers find that by adding pregabalin (Lyrica) to an opiate painkiller, they can get by with half the painkiller dose, thus dealing with tolerance and side-effect risks at the same time.

Drugs which are multi-purpose can be helpful here. Let me use tramadol as a good example. Tramadol is essentially a (weak) opiate, SNRI and NMDA antagonist in one. As anything which activates your μ (*mu*) opioid receptors also boosts dopamine, you have a fairly broad spectrum antidepressant and pain reliever in one. Or the abovementioned pregabalin, which for some people, is like a painkiller, anxiolytic and sleep aid in one.

Benzos can be useful in this sense. Again, to use pain relief as an example, benzos are sometimes good potentiators of pain-relief because they can remove the agitation which can cause an opioid-dependent patient to re-dose more quickly than they would otherwise do. The other useful property of benzos is that they can treat back pain involving back muscle spasms or muscle tension.

Without wanting to sound overly dramatic, a benzo, when used to treat severe, chronic anxiety, is more often than not, a friend for life. A person who has been on a high dose for several decades will find the process of withdrawing to be not only a kind of hell which is almost exquisite in its torture, it can be life-threatening without a very, very, very slow taper. The good news is that when the benzo is a lifelong medication, the issue of tapering is moot.

Finally I wanted to quickly assuage one of the most common concerns I hear. Some people resist benzo treatment because they are concerned with feeling lethargic or "dopey" all the time. Most imagine life on a benzo as one long stretch of feeling "out of it". One of the most attractive aspects of this class is that you build tolerance to the sleepy effects very quickly, however not to the anxiolytic effects. So after a week or so, you will still feel less anxious, however the benzo just fades into the background where it belongs.

Alprazolam (Xanax)

Alprazolam is one of the most widely known and certainly the most prescribed of all the benzos, however everyone knows it by its brand name – Xanax.

Alprazolam is the most potent and short acting of the commonly available benzos and is therefore mostly used for severe panic disorder or for acute anxiety. An important point to make is that one of the reasons why alprazolam tends to be abused more than other benzos is that it can often be more euphoric.

By comparison, most other benzos are fairly mood-neutral or they only improve mood by removing anxiety (If someone is experiencing severe anxiety, they may perceive any benzo as rather euphoric as there are few better feelings than having severe anxiety quelled). This is a double edged sword with alprazolam as the mood-boosting aspects increase abuse, however this property can be extremely helpful in treating someone with anxious depression short term. Longer term, all benzos typically worsen mood, so long term treatment should be avoided where possible.

As mentioned earlier in the book, a drug's addictiveness is typically assessed using three main criteria. A drug becomes more addictive –

- the quicker it comes on (this is why injected drugs are the most dangerously addictive)
- the shorter the duration of effects (a quick comedown encourage re-dosing
- the more potent it is (so alprazolam is believed to be more addictive than, say, lorazepam
- the more it boosts dopamine (which is why opioids and stimulants are addictive)

While there is debate as to whether alprazolam increases dopamine levels, it certainly ticks the first three boxes, so caution should be exercised. Except in the rarest of cases such as severe anxiety disorders, alprazolam should only be used for the short term, as it can be highly addictive for some. If you have any history of substance abuse or addictive behaviours, your doctor will probably not be comfortable in prescribing alprazolam and will look to an alternative with a longer half-life[29].

Recently, in some countries, alprazolam has been re-classified in a more "serious" category compared to the other benzodiazepines due to its popularity as a recreational drug. As well as being the most prescribed benzo, alprazolam also holds the less-appealing title of "most abused" benzo. It is valued by heroin addicts for its ability to reduce the irritability of opiate withdrawal. As a consequence, for relatively short-acting effects, many doctors now prefer lorazepam.

However to reiterate my earlier point, alprazolam is far from being "evil" as some have said. There is more than just a small amount of hysteria surrounding this drug at the moment, which is a shame to the extent that for some people it can be an astoundingly effective drug. I would guess that there are hundreds of thousands of people around the world who owe their quality of life to alprazolam, among the millions helped by the overall class. Ironically, I would also hazard a guess that this number far outweighs those who abuse it.

If you have severe, disabling anxiety which has not responded to SSRIs or other antidepressant-style options, alprazolam could be the difference between being bedridden and having the quality of life you deserve. Similar to one or two other options mentioned in this book, think of alprazolam as your "in case of emergency break glass" option when all else has failed. By "all else" I also mean other benzos. Due to alprazolam's relatively short duration of action, re-dosing can be inconvenient compared to alternatives like clonazepam which can usually be dosed once per day[30]. Just ensure you keep the dose as low as humanly possible and whatever you do, please don't be tempted to take more than what is prescribed to you.

Clonazepam (Klonopin)

Clonazepam is, for the most part, very similar to alprazolam and the other benzodiazepines, however with one key difference – an extremely long half-life. Whereas alprazolam takes effect quickly and works for a few hours, clonazepam can have a half-life of over 24-36 hours. This means that a single dose can theoretically still be effective several days after ingestion, depending on how it is metabolised.

It is therefore used for more long term treatment of severe anxiety disorders such as generalised anxiety disorder (GAD). It is not particularly useful for acute episodes

---

[29] In most cases with drugs of addiction, the faster acting a drug is, the more addictive it tends to be. For example, this is why someone addicted to heroin (which is not only fast acting, but also tends to be injected, further hastening the onset) will be switched to methadone or buprenorphine, which are both extremely long acting and take quite a while to take effect.

[30] In some markets there is a long-acting form of alprazolam available.

of panic or anxiety due to delayed onset of action and long half-life. For sever panic disorder which is episodic and not daily, alprazolam is usually preferred.

If you have been prescribed clonazepam for medium or long-term therapy, you may find that you feel unpleasantly lethargic when first starting treatment. This usually goes away as your body gets used to the drug. As mentioned before, one of the best aspects of benzos for treating anxiety disorders is that you quickly build a tolerance to the sleep-promoting aspects, yet retain the beneficial anti-anxiety effects.

Along with a handful of other benzos (including alprazolam), clonazepam is considered as one of the most potent of the commonly available examples. For instance, 0.5mg of clonazepam = around 10mg of diazepam. Please keep this in mind when using for the first time, if you have been used to taking the weaker benzos.

Diazepam (Valium)

No other benzo can claim the degree of brand-name recognition as Valium, with (frankly, quite scary) huge numbers of housewives relying on it through the 1980s and 90s. It was the highest-selling drug in the US, from 1968-1982, a fact which would no doubt shock the medicine or pharmacology graduate today. It almost seems absurd that for almost 15 years, a powerful benzo like Valium could outsell everything else. Fortunately these doctors are much more cautious, now preferring to reserve benzos for cases truly warranting such a powerful anxiolytic.

Diazepam is another benzodiazepine with a long half-life, so is often used in similar circumstances to clonazepam. Diazepam however, is considered a comparatively dirty drug, with a less selective action and wider range of side-effects. By "dirty", it doesn't mean that it is necessarily "bad" or dangerous. "Dirty" just means that it affects a range of different receptors, which can sometimes create issues if there is an unintended consequence. Amitriptyline and tramadol are other examples of dirty drugs, due to their lack of specificity.

Therefore, while some people may respond better to diazepam than other options, in most cases you are more likely to be prescribed clonazepam if a long half-life drug is warranted.

Lorazepam (Ativan)

Lorazepam is most notable as an intermediate half-life benzodiazepine, so when a half-life somewhere between alprazolam and clonazepam is required, lorazepam is often used. The long half-life of lorazepam is due to its slightly different pharmacokinetics (compared to other benzos), as it is highly protein-bound and not particularly fat soluble. This means it takes longer to reach peak effects and remains effective for an extended duration.

Like alprazolam and clonazepam, lorazepam is a potent benzo, often requiring less than a milligram to be effective.

The main benefit of lorazepam is it tends to cause less of a "drugged" feeling compared to alprazolam in my experience. It is for these reason that lorazepam is now being prescribed more often, as doctors become increasingly concerned about the addictive nature of alprazolam. For what it's worth, I don't particularly subscribe to the placement of alprazolam in its own special "Highly Addictive!" category. The only different between lorazepam and alprazolam is their length of duration and the time they take to start working.

I am actually quite a fan of lorazepam as a happy medium between the recently-shunned alprazolam and the longer half-life benzos such as clonazepam and diazepam. All side-effects (and therapeutic effects) are virtually the same as the other benzodiazepines.

Other benzos

The abovementioned benzos tend to form the vast majority of all benzo prescriptions, however there are many more forms available, depending on which country you live in. For example, during a discussion with a Japanese pharmacist, he said that one of the most widely-used benzos there was etizolam (Depas), which isn't even available in Australia or the US. This was reinforced when I was talking to an old friend from Japan who just so happens to suffer from rather crippling anxiety. She said she couldn't function without "her Depas" and had never even heard of alprazolam or the brand name Xanax. Interestingly, etizolam is the only benzo which adversely affects sex drive – I assume due to its ability to raise prolactin levels, like SSRIs.

Some of the other benzos used include –

Oxazepam –   An intermediate half-life (around 10 hours) benzo

Temazepam –   Another intermediate half-life benzo with relatively mild potency. It tends to be reserved for insomnia and is rarely used purely as an anxiolytic.

Flunitrazepam -   You probably haven't heard of flunitrazepam but I have a strong feeling you would have heard its brand name – Rohypnol – as the infamous "date-rape" drug, where it is supposedly used due to its strong amnesia-inducing effects. Whilst this is largely an urban myth (not even 1% of confirmed data-rape incidents actually involved Rohypnol. This drug is purely reserved for cases of severe, intractable insomnia, almost never used as an anxiolytic.

Triazolam -   Also known as Halcion, this is another benzo used mainly for insomnia treatment as a hypnotic drug. Triazolam, along with alprazolam, is a favourite amongst drug-abusers in countries where it is available.

Midazolam -   An extremely short-acting benzo used mainly in a surgical context or occasionally for severe insomnia.

Chlordiazepoxide -   Known by the brand name Librium, this was the first benzo ever discovered. Whilst we should extend our thanks to Librium for enabling the drugs which followed, it was replaced by far superior benzos. This means that in most countries it has become pharmaceutically extinct.

Whilst benzos are a god-send for intense anxiety states and chronic, intractable cases, they clearly come with a range of downsides such as cognitive dysfunction, over-sedation, adversely affected slow-wave sleep, addictiveness (although much less so than is commonly assumed), gradually increasing tolerance and dangerous withdrawal. Fortunately there's more than one way to remove fur from this particular feline, as you probably expected. By now (assuming you have read the entire book to this point and haven't skimmed, trying to find where it actually gets interesting[31]) you will be more knowledgeable about psychopharmacology than many doctors I have met.

So let's now have a look at some other ways you can treat anxiety by ramping up GABA-ergic activity.

Baclofen (Lioresal)

While it is unlikely to ever be the first-line option when you are looking for anxiety relief, I still wanted to briefly mention baclofen, which is a drug mainly used to treat muscle spasticity in conditions such as multiple sclerosis. Like benzos, baclofen is a GABA agonist, however whereas benzodiazepines broadly target the BzR sub-unit of $GABA_A$, baclofen's action is focused on $GABA_B$, where it acts as an agonist, leading to slightly different subjective effects.

Baclofen is often overlooked by psychiatrists (with most GPs/primary care doctors barely acknowledging its anxiolytic effects), as it is well established that $GABA_A$ tends to be more closely associated with anxiety, whereas $GABA_B$ mainly mediates muscle tension and spasticity. However this fails to take into account a principle I covered earlier, which means that for many people with anxiety disorders, if they are able to induce physical relaxation, psychological relaxation often follows, breaking the vicious cycle which is such a central part of anxiety disorders. Muscles effectively stripped of excess tension can act as a powerful trigger for the relaxation response. In this sense, baclofen works like a pharmacological short cut for non-drug relaxation techniques such as progressive muscle relaxation. Also, one of the advantages of baclofen over benzos is that tolerance generally builds more slowly, as baclofen also has some anti-glutamate effects (more on drugs which affect glutamate in a moment).

While it is clear that for most people, baclofen effectively stops anxiety in its tracks, whether it does so purely as a secondary effect to the muscle relaxation or whether it directly treats anxiety via $GABA_B$, independent of physical relaxation. To use a hypothetical example to explain what I mean, there is debate around whether

---

[31] Spoiler – It doesn't. This is as good as it gets. I'm trying, however the topic of anxiolytics is not exactly a barrel of monkeys…

baclofen would be anxiolytic in the unfortunate event that you wind up as a disembodied brain in a jar, suffering not from muscle tension, but from the rather inconvenient lack of muscles per se. From my experience talking to patients who take baclofen, I get the clear sense that there is at least *some* anxiolysis which is independent of muscle relaxation.

That said, there are some specialists who use baclofen as one of their "go-to" options for treating stubborn anxiety which has not responded to more conventional drugs, because occasionally the results can be spectacular. While baclofen can sometimes be very effective, it is generally perceived by GPs as a "muscle spasticity drug" which happens to have anxiolytic properties through its haphazard activity on $GABA_B$. This can unfortunately mean that not only are many doctors unlikely to think of it as a potential back-up option, many will refuse to even consider it if you were to make the suggestion.

If we look to the horizon, I am hopeful that in the future we may see more drugs which treat anxiety via this pathway, but with more specificity for the neural underpinnings of anxiety. For example, in some research I found in the process of compiling this book, compared to agonists such as baclofen, drugs which acted as *positive allosteric modulators* of $GABA_B$ were far more anxiolytic. In fact, at present there is a huge amount of research going into compounds which act as positive allosteric modulators of various brain receptors, as this mechanism of action is associated with some advantages over traditional agonists and antagonists.

Baclofen also has some theoretical advantages over benzos, as it possesses some of the same effects as *gamma-hydroxybutyric acid* (GHB - more on this later), potentially improving dopaminergic and serotonergic activity. It is this activity on dopamine which sees baclofen being particularly popular with those suffering from social anxiety. However where there's dopamine, there's recreational use, with some users abusing baclofen for this rather unpredictable dopamine kick. Among recreational users, feedback varies from extremely positive to extremely awful. This is echoed with those using it appropriately, with the usual range of *"this drug has changed my life for the better"* through to *"I fail to understand what people see in this useless drug"*.

However it is not all good news. Baclofen is no angel – particularly when it comes time to stop taking it, as it shares many of the downsides of benzos. Most notable of these is its similarly severe withdrawal syndrome after prolonged or high-dose use, with baclofen associated with the same risks around the potential for life-threatening seizures, if it is not tapered carefully and slowly. With baclofen's potent action on the receptors which mediate the muscular component of seizures, particular care should be taken when stopping, and it should never, ever be stopped cold-turkey.

In another one of those strange situations where a compound which is clearly a drug is available as a supplement, there is actually a Russian-developed close relation of baclofen called *Phenibut* (or *β-phenyl-γ-aminobutyric acid*, for those with too much time on their hands) which is available in the USA and other countries OTC. Phenibut is particularly popular in the nootropics community as a kind of anomaly, where you are surprised to find out that a powerful drug is available OTC without a prescription. To be honest, I am not sure why, as Phenibut should not be so freely available. As a result, quite a few people have taken Phenibut at high-ish doses for an extended period, as it is associated with impractically quick tolerance build-up, and then found that the withdrawal effects rival benzos and baclofen for sheer ghastliness.

Please stay away from Phenibut. Not because it is inherently more dangerous than other drugs, but because there are no controls over the production, creating the potential for inconsistent batching or inconsistent potency from supplier to supplier. GABA is not something to be messed with without expert help. However my main problem with phenibut is that people can buy it with their vitamins or supplements without a script, creating the very real possibility of serious harm. After all, if you thought it in a health-food store there is nothing to worry about right? If you still have any doubts, type phenibut + withdrawal into your search engine, where you will hear endless horror stories from those suffering the consequences of misunderstanding phenibut and its potency. In case you needed extra motivation, in some countries where Phenibut is banned, overzealous customs officials and law-makers take a dim view of those who purchase it online through the mail[32].

If you want a safe, effective and legal drug, do just that – start taking a safe, effective and legal drug. Likewise, if you want a supplement which is safe and effective, take a *supplement* (not a drug) which is safe and effective.

To reiterate, my issue with phenibut is around how it is scheduled in certain countries, not with the drug per se. If phenibut becomes a controlled, scheduled drug which is prescribed by doctors, it would become just another GABA-ergic drug in this section of the book. Phenibut is just another gabapentinoid (a modified form of GABA which is able to cross the blood-brain barrier). Fortunately, if you need a legitimate gabapentinoid which is prescribed by doctors, look no further than…

Pregabalin (Lyrica) & Gabapentin (Neurontin)

Both pregabalin and gabapentin were originally developed as anticonvulsants, but were soon found to be highly effective for both anxiety disorders and fibromyalgia, despite being only modestly effective anticonvulsants. Pregabalin is essentially the "updated" version of gabapentin, with increased potency and effectiveness (with some exceptions), much like the way escitalopram is an update on citalopram.

---

[32] To their credit, the more reputable online supplement vendors will not ship Phenibut to countries where it is banned.

These drugs work by inhibiting one of the ways by which your body sends nerve signals around the body and brain, and by reducing levels of excitatory neurotransmitters such as glutamate, substance P and norepinephrine. Patients are often confused by these drugs as the official marketing information clearly states that despite both being a slightly altered form of GABA (not to mention the fact that "gaba" is in their names) and having similar effects on anxiety as do the various benzos, officially they have no direct effect on levels of GABA. However this is actually a little bit disingenuous by Pfizer, as they know perfectly well that pregabalin's pharmacology is clearly going to boost GABA-ergic activity. Due to the yin/yang relationship of GABA and glutamate I mentioned earlier, pregabalin's dampening down of glutamate is naturally going to have the ultimate effect of increased GABA activity.

When we look at pregabalin's effects, the pro-GABA aspect becomes even clearer. Pregabalin boosts an enzyme known as *glutamate decarboxylase* which synthesises GABA from glutamate, while also ramping up the system which transports GABA across neuronal membranes. Both pregabalin and gabapentin are (rather unsurprisingly) gabapentinoids, which are essentially forms of GABA which have slight molecular tweaks to produce unique effects – just like phenibut. Apart from the fact that they are doctor-prescribed, controlled substances, they have significantly more research behind them (even if we discount the Pfizer-funded studies).

In my experience, for mild to moderate anxiety, pregabalin is often the most effective drug available, with none of the problems associated with benzodiazepine drugs such as impaired sleep quality. In fact, pregabalin is also one of the most effective sleep aids available, increasing slow wave sleep, leading to more refreshing sleep quality. In terms of commonly available, mainstream drugs, I could probably count with one hand the number of drugs which increase slow wave sleep.

However these drugs are not without their problems. Due to the fact that they suppress brain activity, they can sometimes have negative effects on cognition and memory. In fact, neurontin is often referred to as '*morontin*' by those taking it, due to the effects on thinking and memory recall. Also, these medications are often difficult to stop, like most other psychotropic medications. This is worth highlighting with reference again to their "supplement" cousin. They potentially have withdrawal effects just as unpleasant as phenibut. If you type in "pregabalin + withdrawal", I am sure you will uncover similar horror stories. The difference is that they are clearly marketed and dispensed as "drugs", not "supplements", so patients are able to begin the process eyes wide open. There is no confusing pregabalin with a supplement.

The other downside of pregabalin is that it is still covered by patent, so it is comparatively expensive. If you do not have appropriate insurance coverage, gabapentin can be a much cheaper option. Although strangely, in Australia, as long as your doctor arranges a special approval via the PBS, pregabalin will be cheaper, as gabapentin is not listed on the PBS. This potentially highlights one motivation which leads some to seek out phenibut, as it tends to be cheaper in countries where neither pregabalin nor gabapentin comes under any government subsidy.

Frankly I continue to be amazed at how few GPs even know that pregabalin is an effective treatment for certain types of anxiety. They would have prescribed it many times for neuropathic pain conditions, not knowing that its usefulness extends far beyond that. This is not an off-label or experimental option, but a first-line option recommended by many experts and anxiety-related governing organisations. For example guidelines published in the *International Journal of Psychiatry in Clinical Practice* (2012) by the World Federation of Biological Psychiatry stated that -

> *"Selective serotonin reuptake inhibitors (SSRIs), serotonin-norepinephrine reuptake inhibitors (SNRIs), and **pregabalin** are recommended as firstline drugs due to their favorable risk-benefit ratio, with some differentiation regarding the various anxiety disorders"*

Then, talking specifically about pregabalin –

> *"The calcium channel modulator pregabalin has been found to be effective in GAD. The anxiolytic effects of the drug are attributed to its binding at the α2- δ-subunit protein of voltage-gated calcium channels in central nervous system tissues. Such binding reduces calcium influx at nerve terminals and modulates the release of neurotransmitters. The main side effects include dizziness and somnolence. The onset of efficacy occurs in the first days of treatment, which is an advantage over treatment with antidepressants."*

Due to the fact that these gabapentinoids are often poorly understood by GPs, it may be worth proactively mentioning them when deciding on your treatment. This is another reason to seek out an experienced psychiatrist as most doctors would never even think of these drugs as a treatment for anxiety disorders. This is strange as they can generate the same kinds of benefits as benzodiazepines but with a far greater safety profile and a relative lack of addictiveness.

If you suffer from anxiety and either fibromyalgia or another neuropathic pain condition, pregabalin may be an extremely effective way of hitting two birds with one stone. These drugs are like dimmer-switches on overactive brain activity, dampening down the frenetic neurotransmission often associated with anxiety disorders. A bonus effect for those with pain who are taking opioid drugs is the fact that pregabalin potentiates the effects of painkillers, potentially allowing you to reduce your dose. I have sometimes recommended the pregabalin/tramadol combination for this reason.

The main problems associated with pregabalin and gabapentin are dizziness and weight gain. Another problem is the rapid development of tolerance, requiring increasing dosages to achieve the same result.

Many doctors are confused by these drugs as they appear to act like mild pain-killing benzodiazepines, yet have no direct action on GABA. This is due to the yin/yang effect of GABA and glutamate I mentioned earlier, which means that there are two ways you can boost GABA – directly boosting it or suppressing glutamate. These two drugs achieve this via the latter mechanism which is why they boost GABA without directly affecting GABA levels or GABA receptors.

Bizarrely, I think pregabalin is a much better anxiolytic than painkiller, with just about every patient I have spoken to indicating that they saw not reduction in pain levels. This is because pregabalin targets a very specific nociceptive (pain sensing) pathway, where malfunctioning nerves send a faulty signal that pain is present

Topiramate (Topamax)

I will only cover topiramate briefly as it is not widely used in anxiety disorders, nor does it have particularly compelling clinical trial data supporting its use. Topiramate is another GABA-ergic drug with a mechanism of action which reads like a combination of baclofen and pregabalin. It should therefore come as no surprise to note that it is mainly used in seizure-related disorders such as epilepsy.

The only anxiety disorder which appears to be benefited by topiramate is PTSD, with at least one trial reaching a fairly positive conclusion regarding its effectiveness. Despite the lack of clinical trial data, I was able to find quite a few anecdotes on various anxiety-related forums. This is yet another drug in the *"I couldn't feel any effects whatsoever"* category on these forums. Topiramate had some fairly negative comments, along with others who have found it astoundingly effective at treating a range of anxiety disorders.

Topiramate does however have one surprising benefit – it appears to trigger weight loss. It is for this reason that lately it is getting used in combination with phentermine to help obese patients lose weight. Why this is interesting is that anxiolytic drugs are almost never pro-weight loss. Drugs which increases the rate at which you burn calories or those that suppress appetite are usually anxiogenic as they make your engine rev harder, whereas the treatment of anxiety usually requires a drug which takes your foot off the gas. In effect, this aspect of topiramate creates a specific opportunity. One of the most common reasons for patients to stop taking their psychotropic medication is unwanted weight gain. This can sometimes be frustrating for doctor and patient alike when the drug in question was successfully treating the anxiety. So topiramate could be a useful add-on to your medication regime if this was applicable in your case.

This category has buspirone as its sole inhabitant, as it falls into the existing cracks of psychotropic drug categorisation. Naturally, buspirone is not the only drug which reduces the symptoms of anxiety by modulating serotonin, as is evidenced by the already-covered SSRIs and receptor antagonists. Or they share buspirone's method of action in addition to SSRI properties, in the case of vilazodone. However as buspirone is free of reuptake inhibition or serotonin receptor antagonism, it tends to have distinct effects which warrant the creation of its very own category.

Buspirone (Buspar)

Buspirone is a fascinating drug which is essentially unrelated to any other drug. It primarily functions as a serotonin receptor (5-ht$_{1A}$) partial agonist, and in certain parts of the brain such as the hippocampus, acts as a full agonist. Partial agonists have quite complicated pharmacology as they activate serotonin receptors when there is a lack of serotonin, yet block the action of serotonin when there is too much floating around the synapse. In addition, buspirone acts as an antagonist of certain dopamine and adrenal receptors, which creates a rather pharmacologically complex net effect on dopamine. This is because activation of 5-ht1A typically triggers the release of dopamine.

Whilst the drugs we have available today are far from perfect, the existence of drugs like buspirone gives me confidence that we can continue to develop increasingly selective drugs with improved efficacy. Because buspirone targets anxiety with laser-like precision, without all the other effects of benzos, it has been called an *anxioselective* drug.

The most important point to note is that buspirone is one of the only dedicated anxiolytics which has no direct effects on GABA. As I have mentioned earlier, while benzos are fantastically effective drugs, GABA (like dopamine as well) can be problematic to the extent that its ubiquity means that GABA-ergic drugs tend to affect many other systems as well as anxiety. Not to mention GABA-ergic drugs like benzos are associated with tolerance and (rare) addictive behaviours. As it has a mechanism of action which doesn't involve GABA, it is free of all the negative effects seen with benzos.

However, like all psychotropic medications, many people report that buspirone was completely ineffective. A common piece of feedback I have heard is that buspirone is "no better than a sugar pill". I think the reason that this is a common reaction is because of buspirone's amazingly benign side-effect profile, with mild dizziness and sedation being the main offenders. However for many people, they experience absolutely nothing – good or bad. Despite this, buspirone is in the "if it works, it really, really works!" category, with many patients reporting that it is by far the most effective drug for anxiety they have tried.

Most would agree however that buspirone is most suited to mild to moderate anxiety, as it is unlikely to be sufficient for the treatment of more severe cases. What this means is that a potential strategy could be to first turn to buspirone, and if it doesn't work, then alternatives like SSRIs and benzos could be considered.

In terms of safety, buspirone is exceptionally benign, however one thing to bear in mind is that grapefruit juice significantly increases the potency and effects of buspirone, so should be avoided.

I have to admit that I have always found buspirone a little perplexing. There are conflicting views as to whether it increases or decreases serotonergic activity, and quite often it fails to elicit any effects (either positive or negative) in many patients.

As I mentioned earlier, unfortunately it is not simply a case of *"reducing noradrenaline and your anxiety fades away"*, as this ultimately depends on *what* exactly is causing your anxiety. For example, depending on both the individual and the context, boosting noradrenaline can often give someone focus and confidence, which can then in turn reduce the psychological component of anxiety. Or, more conventionally, runaway noradrenaline (and adrenaline) can be the source of immense anxiety.

Noradrenaline is a great example of the need to clearly establish whether your anxiety is primarily psychological or physiological. However this becomes complicated when physiological anxiety (such as rapid heart race, dry mouth etc) triggers psychological anxiety. A few years back when I had a public speaking phobia, this was my main issue as it originally appeared out of nowhere. The first few times it happened I would be looking forward to my speech (as a child I was a fairly precocious attention seeker who loved getting up in front of large groups of people to make them laugh) and then be caught off guard by a sudden jump in heart rate and all the other physical symptoms of anxiety. I would then freak out, thinking I must have looked foolish, turning my physical anxiety into psychological anxiety and so on, in a vicious cycle.

So to use the public speaking example, it is helpful to know whether the anxiety is primarily in your body or in your mind as this can dictate how you treat it pharmacologically. If there is a significant anxiety component, where you panic in the days leading up to the event, worried about making a fool out of yourself (which, by the way, most audience members never even notice), a benzodiazepine would be a useful short term Band-Aid. However for others who simply want to kill the physical manifestation of anxiety, drugs which specifically reduce adrenaline and noradrenaline can help. Fortunately, in some cases these drugs can also be rather helpful in treating the anxiety disorders which have a strong physical component.

Beta-blockers

Beta-blockers are an extremely common class of drug used to treat cardiovascular issues such as high blood pressure or an irregular heartbeat. They do this by blocking (antagonising) *beta-adrenal* (β-adrenal) receptors, which control your body's fight or flight response. And considering that an out of control fight or flight response is a central figure in anxiety disorders, they can be incredibly helpful in certain scenarios.

Beta-blockers are particularly helpful where suppressing the symptoms of high adrenaline is required, so they are commonly used by public speakers and even musicians, who could have a performance derailed by shaky hands. To give you an indication of just how effective they are, beta-blockers are banned in the Olympics as they give sportsman who need fine motor control (such as skeet shooters) an unfair advantage.

The best thing about beta-blockers is their safety. Not only are they one of the safest medications available, they are not associated with the same downsides as benzodiazepines, such as addiction or cognitive deficits. However this lack of cognitive side-effects is also a double-edged sword, as they do not have the same ability as benzos to target the psychological aspects of anxiety. They also have no ability to help you sleep; in fact they are associated with worsened sleep quality due to their tendency to suppress the release of melatonin, your brain's "sleep hormone".

In my view, the best use of beta-blockers is in short-circuiting the worrying cycle common in anxiety disorders. By removing the major physical aspects of anxiety, it appears to send a message to your amygdala that it is ok to relax, as the danger has passed. The first time I ever used one for public speaking, I was nothing short of astounded. My cognition was not impaired like it would be with a benzo, yet I *felt* calm and collected. It was then I had a sense of their potential value with anxiety disorders, using my own personal experience.

There are two major types of beta-blockers – non-selective agents and β_1 *receptor*-selective agents. For people with heart-specific issues, selective agents are preferred as they minimize the physical symptoms of fight or flight. However these are just the symptoms we hope to eliminate if we are targeting anxiety, so non-selective agents are preferred. The gold standard beta-blocker in this sense is *propranolol* (Inderal, Deralin).

By far the most interesting application of propranolol in the treatment of anxiety disorders is its use in treating PTSD. One of the major problems with PTSD is that each time the person relives the traumatic event, the amygdala becomes activated, triggering the fight or flight response. This again creates a vicious cycle as each time this happens, the amygdala becomes even more hyper-sensitive and develops a hair trigger. Researchers have found that if you give propranolol to someone immediately after the traumatic event it can prevent the development of PTSD as there is no fight or flight reaction there to help solidify the traumatic memory in your amygdala and hippocampus. Unfortunately however, there is little evidence to suggest that propranolol can reverse PTSD which has fully set in.

Alpha adrenal (α-adrenal) agonists

Alpha agonists have roughly the same physiological effects as beta-blockers, however achieve this via a different mechanism. The alpha-adrenergic receptors in the brain suppress the release of noradrenaline, whereas beta-adrenal receptors essentially have the opposite effect, which is why agonising one and antagonising the other, has very similar outcomes. In my experience, alpha agonists tend to be far more powerful than beta-blockers in killing any noradrenergic activity and have a wider array of uses outside of their main cardiovascular indications.

If propranolol is the gold-standard beta-blocker used to treat anxiety, clonidine is the equivalent alpha agonist. Clonidine is used to treat everything from high blood pressure to opiate withdrawal and even childhood ADHD. If you suffer from the physical side of anxiety, clonidine will effectively stop adrenaline in its tracks. In fact, for some, clonidine is *too* effective, making them incredibly drowsy and even putting them to sleep (however your body acclimatises rapidly, so the sleepiness tends to fade with chronic dosing). Unsurprisingly, clonidine is also an effective sleep aid, which is in contrast to propranolol which can significantly worsen sleep.

With the people I talk to who may benefit from lower levels of noradrenaline, I sometimes suggest they discuss the option of propranolol during the day and/or clonidine in the evening, with their doctor. However clonidine in particular is not to be trifled with. Make no mistake – clonidine is a powerful drug which must be only ever used under expert supervision. You want to slow down a dangerously (or at least *uncomfortably*) high heart rate, not stop your heart altogether.

Alpha-agonists and beta-blockers sit at the intersection of psychiatry and cardiology, so many doctors feel uncomfortable with the idea of what they consider to be "heart medications" being used to treat anxiety. Similarly, some psychiatrists may be hesitant to go down this path, unless they are confident you have no pre-existing heart problems which may be affected. Used properly and by the right people, they can however be incredibly effective, with a much better side-effect profile than most psychotropic drugs. The most valuable role they can potentially play is to enable you to treat your anxiety without resorting to powerful psychotropic medications.

Experimental and "off-label" options

Whenever a drug is approved by the relevant agency in each country (such as the FDA in the USA or the TGA in Australia), it will be approved for certain conditions. For example, pregabalin is usually approved for neuropathic pain conditions, however can also be prescribed to treat anxiety disorders. When drugs are used for conditions unrelated to the "approved" indication, they are considered "off-label". Sometimes people worry that "off-label" implies danger or risk, however in general, drugs are perfectly safe to be used in this way, as long as they are being used for conditions where there is a solid body of experience already. Nobody wants to be a guinea pig and you should be no different.

As well as all the various standard anxiolytics, there are also a few options which can be useful in circumstances where other drugs failed. The main problems with these "off-label" options is that many doctors are not keen to try anything out of the ordinary, despite how compelling the evidence may be. This is both an issue of familiarity and risk avoidance. If your doctor has no experience prescribing a particular drug for a particular condition, often they will be worried about the possible implications for them and their practice. No doctor has ever been sued for malpractice simply for prescribing an SSRI for depression, so unfortunately, you may emerge from the doctor's office with a drug that is not necessarily the best option, but is just the least risky for the doctor. Addressing this and ensuring you get the best possible medication may require either a proactive discussion with your doctor or a referral to a specialist with more experience across a wide number of drugs.

Now I would like to move on to what I believe to be the most exciting development in the treatment of anxiety and depression, perhaps ever (well, at least 20 years).

NMDA antagonists

There is a growing body of evidence showing that one of the most effective potential treatments for both anxiety and depression actually has no direct link to serotonin, dopamine or noradrenaline. That's not to say that there are no effects at all on these neurotransmitters, however this alternative mechanism of action only affects them indirectly, via a downstream mechanism. This pathway to your brain's recovery involves the antagonism of the *n-methyl-d-aspartate* (NMDA) receptor (or, *NMDAR*), which is a major glutamatergic receptor involved in a spectacular number of cellular functions.

One of the first times I heard about NMDAR in this context was a study which sent ripples through the research community. Depressed subjects were given a therapeutic dose of the dissociative anaesthetic *ketamine,* and then found, miraculously, their depression lift within hours. As you might imagine, this is nothing short of astounding. None of the commonly available antidepressants work quickly, with most taking 4-6 weeks to reach full effect. Subsequent research has confirmed that these initial reports were not anomalies, sparking even more studies, as interest in this pathway booms.

According to Professor Colleen Loo, of the Black Dog Institute in Australia –

> "It's truly amazing both in terms of how powerful the effect is, but also how quickly it works. Other treatments we know, medications, psychological therapy, electro-convulsive therapy, take weeks to work. So the fact that you can go from being depressed to being well in one day is unheard of."

Now, this doesn't mean that you should immediately be beating a path to your psychiatrist's door, demanding to be put on ketamine. Despite her enthusiasm, even Professor Loo says that it's "too early to be releasing ketamine for general clinical treatment". More research is definitely required. However the good news is that those first ketamine trials provided the catalyst for research into both better forms of ketamine and other NMDA antagonists. Indeed, the well-known psychopharmacologist I work with recently told me that he was leading a small trial of a proprietary form of ketamine which is administered as a nasal spray to overcome some of the drug's downsides.

This is not an isolated case. As we speak, pharmaceutical companies and other biotechs are busily working on improved ways to take advantage of ketamine's amazing antidepressant effects, as there is considerable enthusiasm amongst researchers regarding this interesting drug. After another study which saw an astounding 75% of people recover from severe, intractable depression after taking ketamine, Melbourne University neuroscientist Associate Professor Graham Barrett was noticeably enthused –

> *"The results are startling," says, who has been studying depression for 30 years. They're not 100 per cent, there are people who don't respond to ketamine, but the results are very, very good."*

The single greatest challenge will be to develop a form of ketamine which can be taken as a tablet. At present, all of these trials require ketamine administered as nasal sprays or regular (and inconvenient) injections. However the good news is that ketamine isn't the only game in town if you want to go down the NMDA antagonism path. More on this in a moment.

So what are NMDARs and why does NMDA antagonism cure anxiety and depression? As I always say, anything to do with the brain is usually more complicated than it seems, and this is particularly the case in this example.

The NMDAR is a type of receptor activated by glutamate, which, as you may recall, is your brain's primary excitatory (or "on switch") neurotransmitter. This receptor is central to just about any synaptic learning which occurs in the brain. As it is so central to everything, when you modulate its activity, it creates a range of downstream effects. As far as we can tell, it is these downstream effects which are important when looking at how this receptor is involved in the pathophysiology of depression. However, we are just at the very beginning of our understanding of this process. Take this extract from a review by the Yale Department of Psychiatry –

> *"Ample evidence indicates that glutamate homeostasis and neurotransmission are disrupted in major depressive disorder; but the nature of this disruption and the mechanisms by which it contributes to the syndrome are unclear. Likewise, the effect of existing anxiolytics on glutamate is unclear, as is the potential of drugs directly targeting glutamatergic neurotransmission to act as novel anxiolytic medications. These are areas of active research. Here we review current knowledge of the contribution of the NMDA receptor, one of the several types of glutamate receptor, to depression and its treatment. Several lines of evidence, in humans and in animal models, support the contention that neurotransmission via the NMDA receptor is dysregulated in depression. Drugs that target the NMDA receptor have shown*

anxiolytic properties in both clinical and preclinical studies. Nevertheless, other effects of such medications, including both cognitive side effects and their psychotomimetic properties, complicate such an application and represent a challenge to the development of clinically useful agents."

As you probably noticed, even the researchers who are right at the cutting edge have an incomplete understanding of exactly why NMDA antagonists treat depression so effectively. However, more and more we are seeing that glutamate, which is affected by NMDA antagonists, is implicated in many different mood disorders. Recall that pregabalin, which reduces levels of glutamate, is an effective treatment for fibromyalgia. In several studies, those suffering from depression were found to have markedly elevated levels of glutamate.

The current best guess we have comes to us via a piece of simple, logical deduction. In addition to the NMDA receptor, another type of receptor for glutamate is known as the AMPA receptor. Wondering what "AMPA" stands for? AMPA is an acronym for *a-amino-3-hydroxy-5-methyl-4-isoxazolepropionic acid*. I bet you regret asking, right? Researchers found that, when subjects were administered ketamine along with an AMPA antagonist (which essentially stops AMPA receptors from being activated), the anxiolytic effects were blocked. This, for me, is compelling evidence which points to the reason why NMDA antagonists treat depression. We have known for a while that suppressing NMDA boosts AMPA, so it appears that AMPA is the key to the antidepressant effect of NMDA antagonists. However it would be simplistic to simply say that the secret to happiness is simply unfettered AMPA activity. What we can say with slightly more confidence is that the level of AMPA activity *relative* to NMDA activity is important.

Again, I will pre-empt your next thought (perhaps with an unwise degree of presumptuousness). Yes, there is already considerable work going into developing drugs which boost the activity of AMPA. Interestingly there are already substances which do this in an approximate way. Known as AMPAkines, or *AMPA positive allosteric modulators*, these substances are widely used in the nootropic community in the form of racetams such as piracetam. Racetams, which are the current darlings of the nootropic community, are great for improving cognition and memory recall, however disappointingly they don't have much evidence supporting their use as anxiolytics.

Researchers are gradually beginning to gain a better understanding of the role glutamate plays in anxiety disorders. And this is not specific to one or two types of anxiety disorders, with glutamate sitting at the heart of just about every form of anxiety, due to its role in fear conditioning. For example, the Cambridge journal *CNS Spectrums* stated that –

"Human clinical drug trials have demonstrated the efficacy of glutamatergic drugs for the treatment of obsessive-compulsive disorder, posttraumatic stress disorder, generalized anxiety disorder, and social phobia."

There is actually one drug already widely used to treat the mood swings associated with bipolar disorder which works by reducing levels of glutamate. This drug, lamotrigine (Lamictal), is also sometimes used in major depressive disorder – particularly with complex or treatment-resistance cases. However unfortunately, despite being effective for bipolar, the general consensus is that it is not particularly effective for unipolar types of depression. This is not particularly surprising when you note that it essentially suppresses glutamate fairly indiscriminately, not distinguishing much between AMPA and NMDA.

However there are some people who have responded well to this drug and I was even able to find a clinical trial for treatment resistant depression which was relatively positive. Like just about anything, if your type of depression or anxiety just happens to be the exact thing lamotrigine treats, you may find it effective. However it certainly isn't the drug which cracks the code of how to modulate glutamate to provide profound relief to a broad cross-section of the community. Unfortunately, when we focus on anxiety alone, apart from some promising results in patients with PTSD, lamotrigine doesn't appear to be particularly efficacious.

To be clear, glutamate is no bad guy. It is one of the most important neurotransmitters in your brain. For readers of Genius in a Bottle (where I extolled the virtues of glutamate in the context of cognition), you actually may be shocked to read about glutamate in this context. Many drugs and supplements which are used to improve memory recall and cognitive processing involve boosting glutamate in some way. However, as with just about everything in the brain, balance is the key, and when glutamate levels are too high for a long enough period of time, some bad stuff starts to occur.

Glutamate plays an absolutely central role in the development and maintenance of anxiety disorders, affecting these neural processes from a range of angles. To give just one example, glutamate is the most important neurotransmitter of *learning from experience*. So if we examine what this means in the context of anxiety and, more specifically, anxiety from an evolutionary standpoint, things become interesting.

Say our hypothetical caveman ancestor walked down a new track and ran into a pride of lions, whereupon he high-tailed it out of there and was able to escape. Using glutamate, your brain would solidify this important information, laying it down as a memory so that you would remember this track and therefore avoid it in the future. Our caveman friend would thereafter feel anxious just thinking about walking down that track.

Glutamate is a double-edged sword in this way. It probably saved our ancestors from being eaten, however due to this glutamate-driven process of memory consolidation, modern day humans can have incredibly difficulty in extinguishing the memory. However in modern day people, dangerous lions and tigers have largely been replaced by an even more dangerous animal – fellow *homo sapiens*.

Actually, even this is too great a simplification. It is not the memory per se, but the connection of the memory with the anxiety it triggered at the time. This is broadly the same principle behind *Pavlov's dog*, where the eponymous Pavlov was able to associate the sound of a dinner bell with food. What this meant was that after repeating the same *paired stimuli* (sound + food) a few times, just hearing the bell would make the dog salivate, even when there was no food in sight. This same concept, when viewed simply from the neurological perspective, is often referred to as *Hebbian learning* (or *Hebbian plasticity*).

So from a research perspective, it appears that by suppressing the activity of NMDA receptors, we may be able to disentangle the bonds between certain innocuous events (speaking in front of a large group of people, driving a car, seeing a stranger walking towards you etc.) and our emotional memory of the event. Or, alternatively, in the case of PTSD, prevent glutamate from making these connections before they have the opportunity to take root.

In addition, from a more direct angle, by suppressing the activity of glutamate, we typically boost levels of GABA, which, as you recall from earlier, is central to the acute process of anxiety. For most people, the "yin/yang" of glutamate and GABA is relatively balanced. However people with certain disorders such as anxiety, fibromyalgia and even Alzheimer's, these two opposing forces fall out of alignment, allowing glutamate to dominate. This is potentially why an already anxious person can accumulate new anxieties and phobias with ease. Their glutamatergic activity becomes out of control, causing you to associate harmless events with some kind of danger. By selectively blocking this process with NMDA antagonists (or other drugs such as pregabalin), we can gradually begin to even up the ledger and put glutamate back in its place.

Chronically elevated levels of glutamate can cause a problem knowns as *excitotoxicity*, which can cause significant neuronal damage and dysfunction. If left unchecked, glutamate becomes a bit like a bull in a china shop, wreaking considerable havoc. To be specific, it is not the glutamate itself which is doing the damage, but calcium, which flows into cells unchecked – kind of like glutamate is holding the door open for calcium. One of the hypotheses regarding the cause of Alzheimer's disease is long term cellular damage caused by excess glutamate. Like patients with depression (albeit in a different part of the brain and to a different extent), Alzheimer's patients typically have extremely high levels of glutamate circulating in their system.

And here's where things get interesting, as a drug used to treat Alzheimer's has recently begun receiving attention as a novel, effective treatment for anxiety and depression.

By now I guess you have read all of this glutamate talk, including the amount of research being done to harness its power as an anxiolytic and thought, *Well this is great, but is there something currently on the market that does something like this?*

Amazingly, there is something which antagonises NMDA to treat anxiety and depression, and you have almost certainly never heard of it. Even if, by some chance you have heard of it, it would be due to its use as a way to slow the progression of Alzheimer's disease.

Memantine is the perfect example of the long lag time it takes for positive research findings to filter down to the patient. Here is a drug with a sizable body of clinical trial data showing it to have powerful antidepressant and anxiolytic effects, backed up by a complex, multi-pronged mechanism of action, yet it remains rarely used as second-line[33] option. In all likelihood, your primary care doctor (GP) will only know of memantine as a treatment for Alzheimer's, and will probably give you a quizzical expression if you ask for it to treat depression or an anxiety disorder. I know this because I have had several people approach me asking for clinical review papers and trial data so that they can convince a sceptical doctor to allow a short trial.

I find this surprising, as, even on paper, memantine's pharmacological profile looks almost too good to be true. Memantine is a complex drug. Anytime you modulate anything related to glutamate, there is going to be a range of secondary effects, due to glutamate's ubiquity in the brain. However let's briefly look at a summary of its main effects -

NMDA and AMPA

I need to get a bit technical here in order to do sufficient justice to memantine's curious pharmacological action. However if this is the kind of thing that makes your eyes glaze over (like my wife, who zones out at the first sign of "brain talk"), just skip the following paragraph.

Memantine is a powerful NMDA antagonist. It is important to note that many of memantine's subsequent effects occur as a kind of chain reaction, triggered initially by the NMDA antagonism. The most obvious effect initially is a boost in AMPA activity, providing a mood boost and improvements in cognitive function.

To continue the "too good to be true", the most interesting aspect of memantine's NMDA antagonism is that it is "non-competitive". This might not sound like much however it is actually quite amazing. Prior to memantine, NMDA antagonists were generally known as being recreational drugs, including ketamine and PCP ("Angel dust"). PCP and ketamine (when taken at recreational doses, which are significantly

---

[33] In most cases, SSRIs will be the initial "first-ling" option. If this fails, the subsequent drugs tried are referred to as "second-line". "Second line" doesn't infer inferiority to SSRIs.

larger than when ketamine is used as an anxiolytic) are actually neurotoxic, or at the very least, not particularly great for your brain. Particularly PCP indiscriminately impairs glutamate function, causing short term cognitive deficits. Memantine however, has the strange ability to only block overactive NMDA activity, leaving most glutamatergic function intact. This is why it is used in Alzheimer's, as it is strongly neuroprotective, blocking the excitotoxicity which damages neurons. To put this another way, memantine only blocks glutamatergic function above a certain threshold, which is why it is perfect for preventing the damage caused by overactive glutamate activity.

So, in effect, what this means is memantine, via its NMDA activity, not only improves mood, but also protects the brain against a common source of chronic, low level neuronal damage.

Dopamine

The next important property of memantine is often completely unknown to doctors, who, if they even know of memantine, tend to think of it purely in terms of its NMDA activity. Memantine is actually also a fairly potent dopamine agonist, with the d2 receptor being the principle target. Whilst your average doctor doesn't typically know this, any neurologist would, because memantine is also used to treat Parkinson's disease and it is the d2 agonism which is key, as this disorder is linked to impaired dopamine function. With reference to this property, memantine is very similar to the other major dopamine agonist used in Parkinson's treatment – pramipexole (Which is also used off-label to treat depression and fibromyalgia). However it should be pointed out that pramipexole, as a dedicated d2 agonist, is significantly more potent in its d2 agonism.

Anything which is an agonist essentially mimics the usual neurotransmitter which activates that receptor, so memantine's d2 agonism functions like extra dopamine availability. This should provide additional mood-boosting effects and contribute to memantine's overall usefulness in treating depression and anxiety. However without wanting to belabour the point, enhancing dopaminergic activity is going to be most helpful in social anxiety, but less so with other types. Indeed, a quick look through the various threads on the Social Anxiety Support Forum online shows that memantine is increasingly being used to treat this condition (with varying degrees of success, naturally).

Serotonin

Memantine also acts as a weak antagonist of serotonin receptor 5ht3a, however it should be pointed that it is unclear to what extent this contributes to any anxiolytic effects. 5ht3 receptor antagonists are typically used as anti-nausea drugs in the treatment of morning sickness or chemotherapy-related nausea.

This highlights an important point to make following on from the summary of mirtazapine from earlier in the book. Some people get confused when they hear of serotonin antagonists treating anxiety and depression – after all, why would blocking the effects of serotonin be a good thing? However there are some receptors which improve mood when agonised and some which do the same when they are blocked (antagonised). 5ht3a is one of these, so, similar to mirtazapine, memantine's antagonism of this receptor may provide some additional antidepressant effect.

To demonstrate, think back to SSRIs, which are well-known for triggering nausea and GI upset in some people. This is because their broad-spectrum activity on serotonin means that they activate 5ht3, which can trigger GI problems. Again, this is why mirtazapine can often be helpful as an add-on to SSRIs, particularly where the depression is also associated with stomach problems. Considering that depression and GI upset tends to go hand in hand, this can be immensely helpful and memantine could potentially be helpful in this regard.

Sigma receptor

The sigma receptor is one of the most mysterious and poorly understood of all receptor types in the brain. However what we do know is that sigma receptor agonism is strongly correlated with improvements in depressive symptoms. It is thought that the SSRIs sertraline and fluvoxamine's sigma agonism contributes to their anxiolytic effects. Just about any pleasurable drug of abuse, such as morphine or amphetamine, also act as sigma receptor agonists. In several rodent trials, memantine has been used specifically as a sigma receptor agonists to quantify or confirm any antidepressant effects. These trials generally concluded that memantine provided a clear mood-boosting effect.

Exactly why sigma receptor agonism should be positive for mood is not fully understood, however the most likely reason is that activating this receptor increases levels of dopamine as a secondary effect.

For those interested in learning the pharmacology of memantine, hopefully the above outline peaks your interest. I want to be clear that, whilst memantine is a great example of a drug rarely recommended by doctors (and even most psychiatrists), it doesn't mean that it is going to be the panacea for all people. Memantine may or may not be of benefit, depending on your particular neurochemistry. In general, the response to memantine can be broken into three outcomes. For some, memantine does absolutely nothing for them. For others, they see a benefit however they cannot tolerate the side effects. Lastly, some people find memantine life changing. These people will often report that they had tried every possible anxiolytic without responding, before finally trying memantine and feeling "cured".

It is also important to point out that, linked to this topic, memantine's side-effects are unpredictable. Most people experience no side-effects once they are through the start-up period (more on this in a moment). Others experience side-effects ranging from minor, through to troubling, through to intolerable. The most common side-effects are –

- Cognitive impairment/memory problems
- "Brain fog", which involves a feeling of disconnected fatigue
- Dizziness
- Sleeping problems, such as insomnia

One of the problems with memantine's side-effects are that they all come on very gradually, over the course of 2-3 days, due to memantine's amazingly long half-life (A single dose can remain effective for 48 hours). With most drugs, you notice the side-effects almost immediately because they come on quickly. If you take something and you get a headache or a stomach ache, it is pretty hard to miss. Memantine's side-effects come on so slowly that they only reach prominence after a few days and there can be a further day or so of lag before someone realises that something is an issue. This is further compounded by memantine's propensity to trigger strange and unusual side-effects which the person has no previous experience of. Everyone knows what a headache feels like however most people have no idea what "brain fog" even means. Brain fog is a bit like the Buddhist and Hindu concept of enlightenment, impervious to any attempts to describe it. All I can say is that, if you get brain fog, you will know it when you see it.

The single greatest downside of memantine is the start-up period. For many people, memantine can be incredibly tough to start, while for others, they experience no issues whatsoever. The most commonly reported problem is this notorious "brain fog". The most likely cause of brain fog is yet another one of memantine's actions. It also acts as a nicotinic acetylcholine receptor antagonist, which is actually a great thing longer term, but at first can be unpleasant. Similar to the difficult SSRI start-up, when you first start memantine it responds by upregulating nicotinic acetylcholine activity, which can be unpleasant. The best way to think of it is like this – imagine a drug that makes you sharper, quicker and with better memory recall. Now imagine the exact opposite of this. That's what starting memantine can feel like for some. The nicotinic acetylcholine receptor is the main target of nicotine (no prizes for guessing this), so by blocking this receptor you are essentially experiencing one of the aspects of why cigarettes are so difficult to quit.

However, once your brain adapts, this is where the magic happens. For some reason, antagonising these receptors eventually leads to heightened activity at these same sites. As major depression can often be associated with cognitive impairment, this can again contribute to a person's recovery and overall mood.

The good news is that all of this unpleasant business can usually be avoided by utilising a careful, conservative and gradual titration period, where you start on a tiny dose and slowly increase. From my experience, I usually recommend starting at no more than 2.5mg, which may involve the purchase of a pill cutter to split 10mg tablets into four. I have heard of some specialists starting their patient on 10mg which I think is crazy and would just be asking for trouble. Unless there was some urgency, increasing the dose in 2.5mg increments per week would usually be sufficient to avoid unpleasant effects.

The final decision that you and your physician need to make is the targeted eventual dose you will be staying on for the duration. There is no hard and fast rule here. Some people get benefit at 10mg, some go as high as 40mg. If you increase the dosage slowly, you should get the opportunity to get a feeling for where your particular sweet spot is. Importantly, the trials which looked at memantine as an anxiolytic or antidepressant generally saw negative or insufficient results unless the dose was higher than 20mg. In general, the sweet spot should be just below the highest dose you are able to tolerate. Whilst you may see sufficient benefit at a lower dose, it is generally those that can tolerate between 20-40mg who see the greatest benefit. This is ultimately an unfortunate aspect of memantine that we can hopefully address with newer, better drugs. I believe that there are a significant number of people who would benefit from memantine however are unable to tolerate it at high enough doses.

The good news is that, while the start-up effects can be unpleasant, they generally resolve within 2-3 days. However whenever you increase your dose, you may be see some adverse effects. This means that, for example, even if you were stable on 10mg for months and then increased to 15mg, you will usually experience the same start-up effects which you saw when you first started.

One final point to make is that, due to memantine's very long half-life, a single dose will remain active for 1-2 days, making the initial start-up period tricky. This is also another reason to go slow. If you suddenly increase from 10mg to 20mg in one day, by the second day you would have accumulated dramatically more memantine. This then means that, due to this long half-life, there will be nothing you can do for the next few days to reduce it. Believe it or not, there are some complete idiots who see that memantine is in the same category of drug as ketamine or PCP and then proceed to ingest huge doses (100mg+). Typically, this then results in 2-3 days of what can only be described as psychedelic hell. Use this as a cautionary tale to ensure that you avoid aggressive dosing or titration schedules.

Tramadol (Ultram)

One of the most common off-label anxiety and depression treatments is the painkiller tramadol. Tramadol is actually structurally similar to venlafaxine and works in a similar way to increase levels of serotonin and norepinephrine. However tramadol also acts on opiate receptors, dulling physical (and psychological) pain, reducing anxiety and lifting mood.

Tramadol is an unusual drug in terms of where exactly it fits and even what it is. There is considerable debate around just about each of its main actions, for example, whether it acts as a serotonin reuptake inhibitor or a serotonin releasing agent; whether it should even be considered an opiate and so on. One of the reasons for this is that tramadol has one of the longest lists of actions of any psychotropic drug. In addition to its main modes of action, it is also a weak NMDA antagonist and also boosts dopamine as a secondary effect caused by its opiate activity.

Tramadol is usually prescribed these days to treat fibromyalgia, where it is extremely effective at giving quality of life. Fibromyalgia patients often mention that, as well as dulling pain and improving mood, tramadol helps to lift the "cognitive fog" associated with the disorder. This cognitive fog can mimic the same type of cognitive dysfunction seen in cases of major depression.

The main downside is that the withdrawal from tramadol (particularly after taking high doses above 400mg per day for long periods) is legendary for its severity. This is primarily due to the fact that while you are withdrawing from tramadol, you are effectively withdrawing from an opiate and an antidepressant at the same time.

Tramadol is also noted for its ability to decrease the seizure threshold at higher doses. However this tends to generally be an issue when someone abuses it. For example, the typical maximum daily dose is 400mg, however I have read stories about people taking 1000mg and having a grand mal seizure.

The other danger of tramadol is the potential for serotonin syndrome. Actually, now is probably a good time to cover this topic as it may save your life one day. If someone combines high doses of multiple drugs which all work on serotonin, there is a chance to develop this deadly condition, which, if you survive it, will at least be the most unpleasant experience you will ever have. However I should point out that it is incredibly rare and in the vast majority of cases, involves a MAOI. This is why you are always instructed to have a break between finishing a MAOI and starting an SSRI (or the other way around). I can't count the number of times I have seen someone on an internet forum experience an unpleasant side-effect of their antidepressant and diagnose themselves with serotonin syndrome. If you did get serotonin syndrome, you wouldn't be telling the tale on an internet forum the next day.

The main reason I wanted to mention serotonin syndrome here is that there is a widespread belief that you cannot combine tramadol with SSRIs or TCAs. While you certainly cannot even consider taking tramadol with a MAOI, the combination of tramadol and SSRIs is surprisingly common. That doesn't mean that it is risk free, just that your psychiatrist or pain doctor needs to assess the risks based on your individual circumstances. If anything, my experience has been that SSRIs appear to block some of tramadol's effects, rather than amplifying them.

Another point which should be noted is that tramadol is converted into its active metabolite by your liver enzymes. Without this conversion, tramadol would possess negligible opiate-like effects. Different people metabolise tramadol in vastly different ways, so this should also be a consideration.

Unfortunately there are few doctors willing to prescribe tramadol off-label for anxiety or depression, despite the large volume of anecdotal reports from people who did not respond to traditional antidepressants yet were seemingly "cured" by tramadol. If you have no quality of life and you have exhausted all options, make sure you discuss off-label options such as tramadol or other medications with your doctor.

One of the other major benefits of tramadol compared to other opiates or benzodiazepines is that tolerance increases much more slowly, allowing you to remain on a small dose for longer. If it weren't for their notorious tolerance issues, opiates could be used more commonly to treat anxiety disorders. Those unfamiliar with the effects of opiates are usually unaware just how effective they are at killing anxiety. However, as tolerance increases over time, you gradually need more to have the same effects and will eventually reach dangerous territory where you could easily overdose and die. In a macabre way, tramadol's seizure risks means that someone would struggle to reach a dose high enough to OD, if at all they could.

If we remove depression and pain from the picture and focus solely on anxiety, I am a little less sold on tramadol. That's not to say that it can't act as an effective anxiolytic. Anything which activates opiate receptors (thereby boosting dopamine also) and increases levels of serotonin is going to have at least some anti-anxiety effects. Tramadol is slightly held back due to its activating and stimulating effects caused by boosting noradrenaline. This can exacerbate anxiety in some.

Finally, it is worth pointing out that recently a new drug which is essentially "Tramadol v2" was released – tapentadol (Palexia). As it is relatively new and as such, most clinical trial data would be linked to the company that developed it, it would be premature to give my view either way. The main difference between tapentadol and tramadol is that the newer drug lacks any serotonergic effects and has a slightly more potent opiate effect. Despite this lack of serotonin effect, tapentadol has demonstrated some efficacy in treating depression, although for this same reason, I can't imagine too many scenarios where it would be prescribed to treat anxiety disorders.

One scenario I can imagine however, is where someone is anxious and in pain and they are already on an SSRI. Many SSRIs block the activity of the liver enzymes needed to convert drugs like tramadol or codeine into their active form. If you took codeine and lacked this enzymatic ability, virtually nothing would happen and your pain would be unchanged. Codeine is actually fairly inert without this process as it needs to be converted in the liver into morphine. This is a fairly common challenge for psychiatrists and pain doctors – particularly as mood disorders and chronic pain are common bedfellows. These doctors often have to choose between switching antidepressants to one that doesn't block these enzymes and moving into stronger opiate territory (morphine, oxycodone etc.) Tapentadol could potentially be valuable here as it doesn't require these same enzymes which tramadol does.

Stimulants

Many people are shocked to learn that, before the advent of modern antidepressants, amphetamines were widely used to treat depression. These people are even more shocked to learn how widely stimulants are still used to this day for the same indication. One of the main stumbling blocks here is actually the word "amphetamine", because of its strong association with street drugs like methamphetamine. If I told you there was a brand new drug on the market called "miraculexatine"[34] which gave you energy, focus and motivation, made you happy and reduced anxiety a couple of hours after taking it for the first time, you would head straight off to the doctor to demand it wouldn't you? For some people, this is exactly what amphetamine does, however there are good reasons why it isn't the first line treatment used by GPs and primary care doctors.

The two main stimulants used to treat mood disorders are the same two used to treat ADHD – dexamphetamine[35] (or variations of, such as Adderall) and methylphenidate (Ritalin). While both of these drugs primarily target dopamine (and noradrenaline to a lesser extent), they work in very different ways.

Dexamphetamine is known as a releasing agent, which basically means that it increases the amount of dopamine, noradrenaline and serotonin (to a much lesser extent) released in your brain. Imagine your brain has a tap through which each neurotransmitter flows. Amphetamines turn the tap to "high", causing the flow to increase. Methylphenidate on the other hand is primarily a dopamine reuptake inhibitor. Think of it like an SSRI for dopamine instead of serotonin. By blocking the reuptake of dopamine, more of it remains in the synapse, thereby leading to improved mood.

If this all sounds too good to be true, that's because it is (with some important exceptions). Anything which boosts dopamine – particularly in the brain's pleasure centres like the *nucleus accumbens* or the VTA – can be addictive for some. For those predisposed, stimulants can be incredibly habit-forming and lead to maladaptive and ultimately destructive behaviours. In addition, these drugs can increase the risk of cardiovascular complications in some people. Finally, a major downside of anything which boosts dopamine is the development of rapid tolerance. This can mean that increasingly large doses are required to achieve the same effect.

---

[34] © Benjamin Kramer 2015 – Just in case!
[35] Also known as *dextroamphetamine*

Unfortunately, for many, their tolerance to the beneficial aspects of amphetamines increases, yet their tolerance to the side-effects doesn't.

Primarily for these reasons, stimulants are these days reserved for treatment resistant depression (TRD), which is where the patient has tried just about everything and still remains depressed. In these cases, amphetamine in particular can be as close as we come to a miracle drug. When I was first researching this book I spoke to all of my contacts in psychopharmacology and was rather surprised to learn just how widely amphetamine is used in these cases. I think this is generally due to a deliberate (and appropriate, in my opinion) effort to avoid publicising this fact. The last thing anyone needs is drug-seeking individuals to be claiming TRD in an effort to gain access to their drug of choice.

However if you are out of options and remain anxious and depressed, don't discount amphetamines as a potentially life-saving option. It is fairly common to see chronically depressed people experience a miraculous improvement soon after beginning treatment. Methylphenidate is less effective, in general, for mood disorders, however for some it can be the best option for them.

Another little-known option is a relatively weak stimulant known as modafinil, which is mainly used to treat narcolepsy or the fatigue associated with sleep apnoea. There is not much evidence supporting its use in mood disorders, however if you are depressed as a result of chronic insomnia, it could be a great option to help you get back on track. I have read the occasional miracle story on an internet forum, so I wouldn't completely discount it for depression, however not for anxiety. Which leads me to my main point.

The link between stimulants and anxiety is a very tricky topic. The general wisdom is that stimulants are not suitable for those with anxiety disorders as they can make things worse. However there are some major exceptions, so if your psychiatrist suggests a stimulant for your chronic anxiety, don't discount it as an option. It all depends on the source of your anxiety. In general, people with social anxiety tend to get amazing benefits from amphetamines, as they usually increase social confidence. These people are often shocked to experience this, as they were initially worried that amphetamines would make them more anxious. Being calmed by amphetamines can be a strange feeling. Or to take a slightly different tack, if you have a form of anxiety which is strongly physiological (racing heart, dry mouth etc.) or concerned with generalised "worry", amphetamines are more likely to make things worse as many of their effects have considerable overlap with the symptoms of anxiety itself. However if your anxiety is linked to a lack of confidence (particularly around groups of people), they can be incredibly effective.

However I should make an important distinction here. These beneficial effects are specific to amphetamines. In all but the rarest of cases, methylphenidate and modafinil are more likely to trigger panic attacks than prevent them.

Barbiturates

By far the vast majority of anxiety disorders can be treated by one or more of the previously mentioned drugs. In fact, when you get down to it, most people are able to settle on an SSRI that works, plus a low dose benzo daily (or as needed when you start the SSRI[36]). However for some people with particularly severe anxiety, genetic issues with metabolism, or with a particular neurochemical makeup, something stronger may be required. Fortunately there are two classes of drugs which, despite their reputation, may work when all else fails.

You know a drug has a PR problem when the only thing most people know about it is that various celebrities such as Marilyn Monroe killed themselves with it. And the people that do know about it tend to view it as obsolete.

Certain parts of the medical profession and the general public were too young to remember the time when barbiturates (barbs) reigned supreme in the treatment of anxiety. Before the advent of newer drugs, in those days if you went to the doctor to discuss problems with sleeping or anxiety, you would be likely to leave their office with a script for barbs. This was a huge challenge because barbs don't play nicely with other depressants such as alcohol. This is where the majority of problems occurred, rather than the patient simply consuming barbs alone.

People nowadays love to bash benzos, however when we look at benzos in the context of barbs, they start to look like a wonder of modern pharmacology. For a start, benzos addressed the awful therapeutic window of benzos, where the difference between a person's recommended dose and the lethal dose having little margin for error when someone is on a high dose. This is why alcohol with benzos has led to so many accidental deaths. When you combine one powerful depressant (alcohol) and another (barbs), you can become so sedated that your breathing slows to the point of death.

All that said, barbs still have a place in modern pharmacotherapy for these stubborn cases. They act in roughly the same way as benzos, activating certain GABA receptors to slow everything down in the brain, including any anxiety. They also suppress the activity of glutamate, creating a "double whammy" effect. It is virtually impossible to feel anxiety while you are on barbs.

Unfortunately however, barbs are known to have the quickest accumulation of tolerance, meaning that more and more of a powerful job is required. Not that you really want to get to this point, as barbs are also legendary for their withdrawal process. Benzos, alcohol and barbs are relatively unique in that their withdrawal can be potentially fatal if not conducted under medical supervision. If you decide to

---

[36] If you have panic disorder or a phobic disorder, you may need to have a benzo on hand for emergencies.

stop a reasonably large barbiturate dose cold turkey, you stand a better than average chance of having a seizure and dying.

This is not a class of drug to be trifled with. However I would deduce that anyone with anxiety severe enough to warrant barbs would need to be on something for the rest of their life, rendering the withdrawal scenario meaningless. I would also deduce that the majority of people taking them do so sensibly. The majority of deaths would be caused by someone abusing them or not being sufficiently warned regarding the various dangerous combinations.

There are a range of barbiturates available in different countries however by far the most commonly known is phenobarbital, which is actually used more commonly treating seizures (Like pregabalin and gabapentin, most treatments for seizures are based on harnessing GABA's ability to sooth hyper-excited neurons).

In summary, the consensus of most medical professionals would be that barbiturates should only be considered as a last resort, due to the risks involved and the fact that superior drugs are now available. Unless you are desperate, they are not going to be much fun. Sure, they will knock you out cold (which, if you have suffered from severe insomnia, will be welcomed), however due to their long half-life you will feel like a zombie the day after.

For 99.99% of the population, barbiturates would be the worst possible option you could consider. However for the remaining 0.01% (actually the figure is probably lower than this even), barbiturates could be the one thing that quells severe, disabling and tortuous anxiety.

Opiates and Opioids

Now we move on from an anxiolytic class with a deservedly extreme reputation (barbiturates) to perhaps one of the most misunderstood drug classes. This is to be expected, as opiates not only have a complex mechanism of action which affects a huge number of brain functions, they are also inextricably linked in the public's mind with addicts injecting heroin and further back, the opium dens of China, which to this day was one of colonial Britain's most shameful acts.

It is beyond the scope of this book to look at the entire subject of opiates in general. There is such hysteria in the media, with talk of a "painkiller epidemic" reaching news headlines on a weekly basis that it would be unwise of me to comment on the global effects of opiates. So I will simply refer to the use of opiates in the treatment of anxiety disorders, in medical terms.

This topic is so complex that I may seem like I am either contradicting myself or changing my mind multiple times over the next few paragraphs, so please bear with me. Perhaps this contradiction is best evidenced by me saying that opiates are probably the single greatest anti-anxiety and anti-stress drug available, yet in my view should almost never be used specifically for this purpose in isolation. By "in isolation" I mean as a treatment for anxiety only. However when there is a combination of intense physical and psychological pain, opiates are without equal. Naturally, the example which springs to mind for most is the treatment of cancer-related pain. No other drug on earth could work as well at relieving suffering in this scenario.

However, aside from this extreme example, chronic non-cancer pain and anxiety tend to be common bedfellows. This is because each one can cause the other. Chronic pain can lead to chronic anxiety due to a range of reasons, however chronic anxiety can also lead to chronic pain. The best example of this is fibromyalgia syndrome (FMS).

Fibromyalgia is still a poorly understood condition, with a range of "causes" and a huge list of symptoms. However the fact that FMS is almost always associated with anxiety and depression points to a strong neurochemical connection. However the problem is that FMS is different for each person, so we can't definitively say that serotonin, noradrenaline or dopamine is behind the condition. To a large extent, this is because FMS is not a singular disease, but a cluster of symptoms which have been given the label "FMS" to enable better treatment of patients. If you have diabetes or Alzheimer's disease there are tests that can be done to definitively show what is wrong. Unfortunately there is no MRI scan or blood test which can prove its existence.

There is one small exception to this, however it is not reliably present in all patients. Some FMS sufferers show heightened reaction to painful stimuli under a brain scan. So, for example, there may be a small pin prick which is so soft that you couldn't even feel it. However for some FMS sufferers, the same amount of pressure will be registered as painful in their brain.

I wanted to cover FMS for a couple of reasons. Firstly, just about every person I know with FMS also has an anxiety disorder of some description. Secondly, even if you don't suffer from FMS, the use of opioids in treating FMS gives us a better understanding of the effects on anxiety disorder.

So why are FMS and anxiety disorders so strongly correlated? I think there are a huge number of individual reasons for this, however there is one theory that I sense would explain many individual cases. FMS is extremely common in people who either had a traumatic childhood which featured constant stress or people who have gone through a traumatic and stressful experience as an adult. One theory which has gained acceptance is that FMS sufferers have a stress response which has been stuck in the "on" position, so their body is constantly at "battle stations". This is one of the reasons why FMS sufferers tend to experience poor quality sleep – when your brain is on the lookout for danger it keeps you from entering into the deeper stages which help you awaken refreshed.

As someone with an anxiety disorder, you may find it helpful to ask yourself this question – Is my brain constantly at DEFCON 1, scanning my surroundings for danger? Sometimes the answer to this is obvious and sometimes it requires a bit of introspection. The challenge then is how to convince your brain that your environment is safe, as it won't simply respond to your command. You may need to do some work on it, consciously noting that you are in a safe, protected space.

Despite the overlap between FMS and anxiety, along with the fact that opiates tend to be powerful anxiolytics, they are not that commonly used to treat this condition. For most people, addressing the serotonin/noradrenaline/dopamine connection tends to bring down pain levels. That's not to say that opiates are never used, they just tend to be reserved for when other FMS medications such as duloxetine, amitriptyline or pregabalin don't provide relief.

By far the most commonly used opioid by doctors treating FMS is tramadol. This is not surprising when you see that tramadol boosts serotonin, noradrenaline and dopamine[37], along with having a mild opiate effect.

So what place do opiates have in the treatment of anxiety? This is a difficult question to answer. Many heroin addicts report that their heroin addiction is a form of self-medicating. You would be shocked at how many heroin addicts and even alcoholics are trying to medicate their own severe and disabling anxiety. However opiates are complicated by their obvious and not so obvious shortcomings –

Tolerance – You will gradually need a higher dose to get the same anxiolytic effect. This compares to most antidepressants which can be taken at the same dose indefinitely[38].

Addictiveness – For a small minority of people, opiates are incredibly addictive. Unfortunately, the more effectively an opiate treats someone's severe anxiety, the more likely they would be to become addicted. In some ways this should not be surprising. Imagine you suffered severe, constant anxiety your whole life and then one day you tried a drug which made you feel "normal". You would probably say that addiction is a small price to pay.

Long term effects - They tend to make you more anxious over time because opiates suppress your stress response. Consequently, many opiate addicts report having terrible stress tolerance and fall apart at the slightest hint of stress.

---

[37] Tramadol boosts dopamine indirectly. When a drug activates your mu-opioid receptors, it triggers dopamine release.
[38] An exception here is when a drug "poops out", requiring a new alternative. However this is not linked to tolerance.

Clearly, the most relevant example in the context of opiates and anxiety is where someone with an anxiety disorder also suffers from severe, debilitating chronic pain. If this describes you, and you are already prescribed an opiate painkiller, you would no doubt be well acquainted with the anti-anxiety effects of these drugs. However what I usually say to people in this situation is that you should only take as much of the drug you need to manage your pain. I don't think it is a good example to increase the dose so that you also treat your anxiety disorder. Try to address the anxiety through other drug-based and non-drug therapies.

What about current research and future drugs on the horizon?

It appears as if researchers are finally emerging from a long-term, blinkered view of anxiety and depression which focused entirely on serotonin. As this view changes, you can expect to gradually see some interesting (and potentially life-saving) drugs hit the market in time.

A large chunk of current research into mood disorders is focused on two main areas of interest[39] –

- The glutamate/GABA system
- The cannabinoid system

Let's have a quick look at each. I want to do this for several reasons. Firstly I want to give hope to those who have not been helped by existing drugs. There are some really interesting, novel options on the horizon. I also wanted to reiterate my point that mood disorders don't begin and end with serotonin and dopamine.

Glutamate/GABA

As explained previously, glutamate and GABA are like the brake and the accelerator. If you want the car to go more slowly, you either take your foot off the accelerator or you press the brakes (Well, actually you should probably be doing both, if you want to be a safe driver!). So, if we acknowledge that this system may be involved in mood disorders, naturally we need to look at both the brakes and the accelerator. Let's use pregabalin (Lyrica) for example. Pregabalin often confuses people because it reduces anxiety and muscle tension in a similar way that benzodiazepines do. However in this example, benzodiazepines are the "brakes" (they activate GABA receptors, slowing down the brain) and pregabalin is "taking your foot off the accelerator" (it reduces glutamate activity, therefore intensifying the

---

[39] Note – Naturally there is research being undertaken looking at other areas, however these are the two major areas of focus.

effects of GABA). This is great for anxiety, but not so great for depression. So naturally, it seems logical to look at how to create the mirror imagine of this process in order to "put your foot on the accelerator".

Just the other day while I was compiling this book, I saw news of a rodent study using a completely new compound which also demonstrated a powerful anxiolytic effect. According to Scott Thompson, Ph.D., and chair of the department of physiology at the *University of Maryland* –

> *"These compounds produced the most dramatic effects in animal studies that we could have hoped for… Our results open up a whole new class of potential anxiolytic medications. We have evidence that these compounds can relieve the devastating symptoms of depression in less than one day, and can do so in a way that limits some of the key disadvantages of current approaches."*

This compound is classified as a GABA-NAM (Or, if you like impressing people with your cleverness - *gamma-amino-butyric acid negative allosteric modulator*). Essentially what this means is that the compound reduces GABA activity, thereby pressing down on your brain's accelerator. If you have ever suffered from a bout of insomnia and visited the doctor, you are likely to leave their office with one of the "Z" drugs such as zopiclone (Lunesta) or zolpidem (Ambien, Stillnox). These drugs are technically known as positive allosteric modulators of GABA, which means that they are basically the opposite of GABA NAMs.

As with anything, GABA-NAMs won't be panacea for all, however, for cases featuring either overactive GABAergic activity or underactive glutamatergic activity, they look incredibly promising. The most interesting aspect of the GABA-NAM mentioned in the above study is the similarity with the ketamine trials, where powerful antidepressant and anxiolytic activity was noticed almost immediately. Clearly, by targeting this general system, we may eventually be able to treat depression more quickly and more effectively than with the currently available SSRIs.

The two other major components of the glutamate/GABA research story are NMDA and AMPA, which I have already covered. This means that at some point in the near future, depending on the results of further clinical trials, we will either have drugs which antagonise NMDA receptors or drugs which directly modulate AMPA. Who knows, we may have both, however I sense that eventually we will have a clearer picture of which pathway is going to be more effective.

Cannabinoid system

If ever you wanted the perfect example of my mantra regarding anxiety and depression being caused by different things in different people, the cannabinoid system is the perfect example. You probably know of this system due to its most famous drug – cannabis (marijuana), which works by modulating the CB1 and CB1 receptors. However in reality, the cannabinoid system is one of the most prominent "system" in the brain, with receptors located literally everywhere. Not only is the cannabinoid system located throughout the brain (and in certain other parts of the body), its function is also incredibly complex. Whereas with glutamate/GABA we can talk in terms of "accelerator" and "brake", the cannabinoid system is not quite as simple to explain.

However for the purposes of this explanation, one of the ways this system acts is actually quite similar to this accelerator/brake analogy. Activating these receptors appears to act as a "brake" on cell firing activity. Interestingly, one of the effects of this is an indirect suppression of glutamatergic firing. As explained earlier, drugs like pregabalin were developed to prevent seizures by suppressing overactive glutamate-driven brain activity. You may have heard of those cases where medical marijuana was able to cure life-long, debilitating seizures in children. When we look at the function of the endo-cannabinoid system from this perspective, it is not hard to see why this may be the case.

What we also know is that, by activating the CB1 and CB2 receptors via cannabis, many people see a reduction in anxiety and an improvement in mood. Another piece of the puzzle is the fact that a drug which does the exact opposite of this (Rimonabant – a CB1 antagonist) was banned due to its unfortunate tendency to make people depressed and anxious (and even suicidal).

Great! I hear you say. *I can just light up a joint and my troubles will just fade away.*

I wish it were that simple. Remember, this system is incredibly complex and its effects are highly user-dependent. If you are someone who smokes marijuana or know people who do, you will almost definitely know that everyone responds to marijuana differently. For some people, marijuana is like a key for a lock in their brain that had until that point been inaccessible. It can act as a powerful anxiolytic, reduce neuropathic pain and boost mood. For other people, it can trigger an intense anxiety attack which can be incredibly unpleasant. Other people have no particular reaction at all and wonder what all the fuss is about. Interestingly, males are significantly more likely to get benefit from cannabis than females. Again this is probably no surprise to most, with cannabis renowned for being enjoyed more by males. This appears to be due to the way certain hormones such as oestrogen interact with THC, the main active ingredient in cannabis.

This also provides a useful segway into the next complication with cannabis. If we were to travel a few hundred years back in time and smoked the natural cannabis growing then, it would have significantly different effects than modern-day cannabis. This is because cannabis has been extensively bred to be high in THC, which is the main active ingredient and the part of the plant responsible for the "high" feeling. However there is a downside to this which you may have heard about.

Before cannabis was bred for high levels of THC, the THC was balanced out by another psychoactive component called cannabidiol (CBD). Here's where things get interesting. THC is pro-psychotic, and this is why smoking marijuana can trigger schizophrenic symptoms in those with a latent heretidary predisposition. CBD is anti-psychotic. As you would have now surmised, originally cannabis had more balanced psychoactive effects, whereas most modern day cannabis is now complicated by unnaturally high THC levels. An exception to this is where cannabis has been decriminalised and a mind-boggling variety of different strains of cannabis is now available to buy legally.

Another complication of THC is that over time, and particularly at high doses, it gradually causes various cognitive deficits and memory problems. Sometimes, when it comes to the brain, you can't have your cake and eat it too (as much as you will want to, if you are high on THC and get the munchies). The process by which THC can treat anxiety and depression in some people by literally "chilling them out", naturally slows down cognition. I have witnessed this first hand with a person I knew who was a heavy pot smoker. He was the most "chilled out" guy I knew – nothing seemed to bother him (except for running out of pot!). However, gradually his speech became slower and he struggled to recall certain words or events.

However, here's where things get interesting. Researchers are now working on drugs which selectively harness the beneficial aspects of THC, without causing cognitive deficits. To give you a sense of the optimism currently held in research circles, here is the abstract from a paper published by The Rockefeller University Laboratory of Neuroendocrinology -

> "Substantial evidence has accumulated implicating a deficit in endocannabinoid in the etiology of depression; accordingly, pharmacological augmentation of endocannabinoid signaling could be a novel target for the pharmacotherapy of depression.

> "Within preclinical models, facilitation of endocannabinoid neurotransmission evokes both anxiolytic and anxiolytic effects. Similar to the actions of conventional anxiolytics, enhancement of endocannabinoid signaling can enhance serotonergic and noradrenergic transmission; increase cellular plasticity and neurotrophin expression (brain growth factor) within the hippocampus; and dampen activity within the neuroendocrine stress axis."

> "Furthermore, limbic endocannabinoid activity is increased by both pharmacological and somatic treatments for depression, and, in turn, appears to contribute to some of the neuroaduptive alterations elicited by these treatments."

> "These preclinical findings support the rationale for the clinical development of agents which inhibit the cellular uptake and/or metabolism of endocannabinoids in the treatment of mood disorders."

It is helpful to note that this paper was published in the field of endocrinology (the study of glands which release hormones). I have recently spent an inordinate amount of time researching this area of study on the potential involvement of the cannabinoid system in mood disorders. What gets me most excited is the relationship between this system and the stress response, as chronic stress is one of the most common triggers for depression or anxiety disorders. And as long as you remain stressed, it is going to be incredibly difficult to recover, no matter which drugs you take.

It is still early days in our understanding of the endocannabinoid system, however it appears as if this system may provide us with a way of directly dampening down the stress response. Here is a great way of looking at this – Chronic stress causes chronically elevated levels of the stress hormone cortisol, which is neurotoxic – particularly for the hippocampus. When people with major depression have their brains scanned, they often show dramatic shrinkage of the hippocampus. As you may recall, one of the reasons why we believe anxiolytics work is that they gradually trigger the regrowth of the hippocampus back to normal size, which then correlates with a person's recovery from depression.

The cannabinoid system offers the promise of a way to prevent this whole cascade in the first place – something that no other drug currently offers. That's why I am excited about this research and what it may bring in time.

Only half the story

You may be surprised to learn that all of the various off-label options I have mentioned are just some of the drugs occasionally used for difficult to treat cases. In my experience I have seen just about every different combination of drugs from different classes imaginable. For example, many find that adding an atypical antipsychotic such as olanzapine or quetiapine can be of immense benefit, while many find these drugs to be unbearable.

This is why working with an experienced specialist is vital. They will have a long clinical experience from which to draw potential options and combinations. It is possible that the drug which works for you is not even mentioned in this book! To this end I am currently setting up a contact email where readers can send in their own experiences, whether using something from this book or something else I haven't mentioned (and can then integrate into the next edition).

What happens when the medication doesn't work or the side-effects are intolerable?

The two major problems associated with anxiolytic treatment are poor response and troubling side-effects. However both of these scenarios have a great number of various options available to increase the chances of remission and recovery.

Unfortunately there is an uncomfortably large proportion of people who don't respond to drugs even after trying several types or classes. This is known as *treatment-resistant depression* (or TRD) and, depending on the doctor, is defined as either no response or incomplete response to traditional antidepressants. However this is not just confined to depression, with *treatment-resistant anxiety* also a potential challenge for psychiatrists and doctors. It is important to highlight the fact that anxiety which doesn't respond to any therapies is incredibly rare. It is also important to make the distinction between acute benefits and chronic benefits when assessing how a patient has responded to certain drug therapies. If we use the opiate example, we may see that a patient can stop anxiety in its tracks with an opiate, however this same opiate then just makes the anxiety worse when it wears off. So acutely, we have something that works, however chronically the opiate is actually making the anxiety disorder worse.

If your anxiety is refractory to a range of treatments, it must become an urgent priority for your psychiatrist to address. Suicide rates in people with refractory anxiety are extremely high. Whether it is via increasingly "off-label" drugs or experimental non-drug therapies, all efforts should be made to alleviate your suffering. In these situations, many of the usual concerns need to be put to one side – at least initially. Addictive or not, a high potency benzodiazepine at a higher dose would typically be highly effective in this scenario. At all times, a patient needs to know the price which must be paid in order to treat their anxiety. So if you have suffered from life-long debilitating anxiety with a poor quality of life, issues of addiction and tolerance will be seen as an acceptable price they are willing to pay.

Linked to this, it is vital that you reach a sound understanding with your psychiatrist as to exactly what constitutes an improvement in your anxiety. For example, if you have a fear of public speaking and then just avoid doing any public speaking, would you consider this as an improvement in your anxiety disorder? A psychiatrist may find a phobic patient who now appears miraculously calm, however the reason they are calm may be that they have just avoided everything they were phobic of.

We also need to acknowledge that for many people, their anxiety disorder is a life-long condition which manifests then disappears at certain points of their life.

If you have experienced no relief from your symptoms despite trying several SSRIs, don't despair as you are not alone. This is an unfortunately common occurrence and shows clearly that no one neurotransmitter is responsible for all depression and in many cases the cause may not even be neurochemical in origin. The good news is that there are a range of options available to you. Depression which is completely and utterly impervious to any forms of treatment is exceedingly rare, so it is often a case of finding what works for you.

In general, if you don't respond to the very first drug (which will almost always be an SSRI), doctors will follow a reasonably similar series of sequential steps as they try to get a response –

- Increase the dose of the current SSRI
- Switch to another SSRI (Note that some doctors may do step 1 and 2 the other way around, with the thinking that side-effects tend to emerge at higher doses, so the better option is to first find one that works at lower doses)
- Switch to another class of anxiolytic – This will depend largely on your symptoms. Some common first steps include mirtazapine, trazodone or bupropion, however this depends on the country. For example, in Australia, trazodone is not available and bupropion is only available to help you quit smoking. If these don't work, doctors will then move to the tricyclics such as amitriptyline or clomipramine. If this doesn't work, they may then move on to MAOIs, however many doctors are no comfortable prescribing MAOIs so may skip this step.
- Augmenting an SSRI with another drug – Some doctors may do this before they abandon SSRIs. For example, mirtazapine is a very popular augmenting drug because it can offset the SSRI effects on sleep and can mitigate SSRI-related sexual dysfunction. Another option could be an atypical anti-psychotic like Abilify (aripiprazole), which can sometimes be effective (however with its own set of side-effects which can be worse than SSRI side effects).
- Adding a benzodiazepine to existing therapies

In addition, there is an "in case of emergency, break glass" option, however this tends to be more for severe depression, rather than anxiety disorders. For people in a deep, dark hole, this misunderstood yet highly effective treatment is electroconvulsive therapy (ECT). You probably imagine someone with electrodes covering their brain, thrashing about as if being electrocuted, however this sight is a thing of the past. Today's ECT is safe and surprisingly gentle. However, ECT is beyond the scope of this guide and certainly beyond my field of expertise. My only point is that, if all else fails and your doctor suggests ECT, please do thorough research before deciding either for or against it. ECT saves lives.

Recently, a new take on this approach has emerged. Called *deep brain stimulation* (DBS), it involves sending an electrical impulse to a specific part of your brain via an implanted *stimulator*. DBS is mainly used in Parkinson's disease or MS to treat movement issues like tremors. However it is now also being used to treat people with anxiety disorders like OCD.

DBS is not a cure per se. However it can give long lasting relief in many cases.

The bad news is that the procedure can be quite daunting for many, as it involves a probe being inserted near your chest and then carefully guided to the target area of your brain, whereupon a tiny stimulator is implanted. Also, as with any surgical procedure, you face a range of risks like infection. The procedure could also cause a new problem while treating the old one.

DBS is firmly in the category of treatments which are really only for those who have not improved after an exhaustive range of orthodox treatments such as medication or CBT.

In terms of pharmaceuticals, there are a range of options. Interestingly, many doctors actually consider your anxiety as "treatment-resistant" after trying multiple SSRIs, so the first step is often looking at tricyclics and then, if that doesn't work, possibly MAOIs. Many doctors are nervous about prescribing MAOIs due to the various dietary restrictions, so will often try a range of alternatives before resorting to this class. However please bear in mind that, although MAOIs may have a bad reputation due to these dietary restrictions (and potential blood pressure problems in the event of accidental consumption of foods containing tyramine), they remain the single most effective class of anxiolytics. I think this is primarily due to the fact that they are able to boost all three major monoamines simultaneously.

What you may find is that there are dramatic differences between doctors in terms of how conservative they are or how "adventurous" they are comfortable getting in order to find you something that works. My general philosophy on this topic is that I would always choose the more adventurous doctor if your depression is not responding to standard treatments. Some doctors resist trying less conservative options due to perceived potential side-effects or even addiction risk. I think those things have to sometimes be put aside when there is a life and death question at stake, depending on the severity of the depression.

For example, for some severely depressed people, drugs like tramadol or even stimulants like Dexedrine and methylphenidate can be the only thing that digs someone out of the deep dark hole they have been living in. There is only a very small percentage of the total population that has addiction problems or substance abuse issues, so to withhold what could sometimes be life-saving medication due to this minority of people would be a tragedy. If this is something which may be relevant in your case, don't be afraid to ask your doctor to give you all the options so you can participate in the decision-making process.

If you are simply bothered by side-effects, the situation is a little easier to rectify. Similarly to TRD, if you are experiencing intolerable side-effects, you can either switch medications or augment with other agents. The key word here is *intolerable* and, as you can imagine, this is a highly subjective thing. One person may be able to put up with quite debilitating side-effects while another cannot.

The most common problem with SSRIs is the way that they can boost serotonin to uncomfortably high levels while suppressing dopamine at the same time. This causes the two most common issues with SSRIs – emotional blunting/anhedonia and sexual dysfunction. Fortunately this can be fixed with a drug that boosts dopamine. Most commonly this will be –

Bupropion (Wellbutrin) – Inhibits the re-uptake of noradrenaline and dopamine (covered earlier already).

Pramipexole (Mirapex) – This is one that many doctors don't use yet, as pramipexole has traditionally been used to treat restless legs (RLS) and Parkinson's disease. Pramipexole is a dopamine agonist (in a similar way to how morphine is an opiate agonist), so can boost dopaminergic activity in certain parts of the brain. Considering one of the main side-effects of pramipexole can be "hypersexuality", you can see why it can sometimes be helpful for SSRI patients. One problems with pramipexole is that it can worsen mood in the first few days as your dopamine system compensates for the drug.

Stimulants – Sometimes the addition of a stimulant to an SSRI can be incredibly effective. This is because by boosting serotonin, dopaminergic function can be suppressed by SSRIs. SSRIs can also cause blunted emotions, which can also be alleviated by stimulants. See above section on stimulants for more information.

It is vital to remember that not all anxiety disorders are caused by problems with serotonin. As James Lee explains brilliantly in his book *Better Living through Neurochemistry*, you have a range of neurotransmitters and neuro-hormones, such as serotonin, dopamine, noradrenaline, glutamate, GABA, endorphins and many more. A problem with any one of these neurotransmitters could cause problems with either depression or anxiety. With your doctor, don't be afraid to do a little detective work to find the source of your problems. This is why I recommend Lee's book, as it details the symptoms of deficiencies in all of these major neurotransmitters, giving you a head start in finding out exactly what is going wrong inside that complex organ sitting inside your skull.

The things I wish all doctors took the time to inform you of

If there is one comment I hear from clients more often than just about anything it would be – *Oh my god, I can't believe my doctor/psychiatrist didn't tell me that!*

I never fail to be surprised at just how little information patients are given when they are started on medications for anxiety and depression. This is a shame, as the pharmaceutical treatment of anxiety is associated with a range of challenges and pitfalls which could easily be addressed with better information from doctors. To that end, I wanted to create a list of some of the most important stuff which you can refer back to if or when required. Some of these points have already been touched upon through this section, however I think that having a discreet list in dot-point form would help solidify some of these concepts. So here is my *"Oh my god, I can't believe my doctor didn't tell me that!"* list -

- When you look up the available information on your new medication (s), which is something I always recommend people to do, there are a few important terms to remember, which will make it easier to understand the information –
    - **Pharmacodynamics** (or *pharmacology*) – How does it act on the brain? Which neurotransmitters are affected?
    - **Pharmacokinetics** – How is the drug metabolised? Does its route of metabolism affect other drugs you may be taking?
    - **Contraindications** – Is the drug safe to take based on other medication conditions I might have? For example, if you had heart problems or very high blood pressure, drugs like dexamphetamine or amitriptyline would be contraindicated.
    - **Half-life** – This is way a drug's duration of action is usually represented. However some people confuse half-life with how long the drug will remain effective after taken. For example, the half-life of alprazolam is around 11 hours, however for most people, it remains effective for a much shorter duration than this.
    - C_{max} – This is how the level of the drug in your system is measured. It is also referred to as *peak-plasma concentration.*
    - T_{max} – This is how long it takes for the drug to reach C_{max} after ingestion. For example, the T_{max} for alprazolam is between 1-2 hours, depending on the person. This is an extremely important bit of information to use along with the drug's half-life to enable you to establish the best time for taking your medication.
- Most drugs (at least in oral form at least) are metabolised either by your liver (hepatic metabolism) or your kidneys (renal metabolism). If you are taking more than one drug and both are metabolised in the liver, it can introduce some challenges in some cases. Most psychotropic drugs are metabolised in the liver by an enzymatic system known as cytochrome P450. This system then has sub-types. For example, fluoxetine (Prozac) is metabolised by

CYP2D6, whereas the antipsychotic drug haloperidol is metabolized via CYP3A4. A drug which is metabolized by one of these sub-types is known as a *substrate*.

- Certain drugs also change the activity of certain P450 sub-types in the following ways –
  - o **Inducers** – These drugs increase the activity of this particular sub-type. So if you are taking a drug which induces CYP2D6 for example, and you are taking another drug metabolized by the same enzyme, the inducer can increase the potency of the second drug. This can, in some circumstances be dangerous. For example, if you are taking an inducer of CYP2D6 such as the steroid dexamethasone, along with an opiate painkiller such as morphine, it could make the morphine much stronger in some cases.
  - o **Inhibitors** – These drugs inhibit this particular sub-type's activity, essentially creating the opposite effect to an inducer. If you take a potent inhibitor of CYP2D6, such as bupropion, it could stop your morphine from working. Or to use a more dangerous example, bupropion could stop your high-blood pressure medication (such as propranolol) from working.
  - o Where things get more complicated however, is where the affected drug is a *pro-drug*. For example, the opiate painkiller codeine is a pro-drug. Codeine itself has no painkilling ability to speak of. However when you take codeine, your P450 enzymes convert it into morphine and norcodeine in the liver. Norcodeine has virtually no painkilling ability. So to use the earlier example, whereas an inducer would increase the effects of morphine, it would decrease the effects of codeine because it causes more of the drug to be metabolised into norcodeine instead of morphine
- Based on the pharmacokinetic properties of the drug, you will be able to establish the right drug and then the best way to take this drug. This can be distilled down to –
  - o Drugs with a long half-life usually take much longer to take effect. So, for example, for someone with panic disorder who needs fast relief, a short half-life benzodiazepine such as alprazolam will usually be more useful than a long half-life version such as clonazepam.
  - o Drugs which have a long half-life are more effective for examples where steady levels are needed. If a drug has a half-life of at least 24 hours, you will only have to take it once per day.
- Your psychiatrist may wish to put you on more than one drug at the same time. They may do this to attack the problem from two different angles, use drugs that synergise well or introduce a second drug to address potential side-effects of the first drug. For example, you may be given a benzo to take while you are first starting an SSRI, to prevent the increase in anxiety which can occur as your brain gets used to the SSRI. Some other examples of combinations include –

- o Pregabalin or a sedating antihistamine (such as promethazine) to increase the effects of opiate painkillers. This allows the doctor to achieve satisfactory results at a lower dose.
  - o Mirtazapine added to an SSRI to mitigate sexual dysfunction
- If finances are a factor and you don't have health insurance which covers medicines, for most classes there are off-patent generic versions which can be significantly cheaper. For example, if an SNRI is needed, duloxetine is still under patent, whereas venlafaxine is not and will usually be significantly cheaper.
- Another great way to save money on medications is by getting a high-dose version which you can then either split or cut in half using an inexpensive pill cutter. For example, if you are prescribed 10mg escitalopram, ask your doctor for the 20mg version so you can halve it.
- If there is one thing I hope I have made clear in this section it is that you should never just settle for a sub-optimal response to your medication. After you have given it a reasonable try (4-6 weeks in some cases), if it isn't working or if the side-effects are troubling, ask your doctor about your available options. There is almost always an alternative option or an additional drug to deal with side-effects.
- If there is something you don't like about the drug you are taking and you want to stop taking it, take enough time to make a considered judgement. Something I have seen time and time again is a patient gradually feeling better and forgetting just how unwell they were before starting the drug. They then stop the drug due to a minor reason, only for the anxiety or depression to return worse than ever, causing them to regret their decision. You need to weigh the relative importance of certain side-effects with the original illness. The most common example of this in my experience is where patients stop their medication due to a drop in libido. The usual comment I hear in this situation is that the patient realises that a drop in libido is a small price to pay when you consider the alternative.
- That said, at risk of sounding like I am contradicting myself, sometimes I see the opposite problem. A patient will respond well to an SSRI but with a lower libido being the result. They will then berate themselves for even considering a low libido to be intolerable. Unfortunately, there are even many doctors and psychiatrists out there who have the same position. I get the sense that some of these doctors view this as almost ungrateful, viewing libido as a low priority in the overall scheme of things and being unhappy with it raised as a problem. Sexual activity forms a key part of who we are and the relationship we have with our partner or spouse. Naturally, the importance of sexual activity varies greatly among individuals, with some patients feeling like a key part of their identity is missing, and others who barely notice their lack of libido. If you are suffering from a low libido and want to do something about it, go back to your doctor to discuss the option to either switch drugs or add a new one to mitigate the anti-sexual aspect of their regime.

- If you are taking a medication which is addictive, builds tolerance or able to be abused, such as a benzodiazepine, opiate or stimulants, there are a range of additional challenges and complications such as –
  - Always start on the lowest dose possible and then gradually work your way up to find the right level. If you are taking a drug which builds tolerance, you want to ensure you are able to continue benefiting from it for as long as possible. The best way to do this is to keep the dose low initially and only increase it if absolutely necessary. That said, if the drug is no longer working at your current dose, talk to your doctor about the potential to increase the dose a little
  - Never, ever allow yourself to view your medication as potentially recreational. For example, if someone is prescribed 10mg morphine, they may be tempted to occasionally take 20mg to get high. Not only will this send your tolerance through the roof, your neurochemistry will be all over the place, making genuine recovery difficult. In addition, if this becomes a regular occurrence, you may run out of your medication before you are able to get your script re-filled.
  - If you have a history of substance abuse which your psychiatrist is not aware of, be upfront about it so they know which drugs may be problematic. Developing a substance abuse problem will make any improvements in your anxiety disorder highly unlikely
  - If you are taking something which can also be recreational, you need to make a subjective assessment regarding the difference between getting high and an improvement in your anxiety symptoms. Knowing where the line is can be rather tricky as there are no simple black and white rules. Say you are prescribed dextroamphetamine for depression and take a single tablet, whereupon your mood brightens an hour or so later – the exact effects your doctor was targeting. Say you then take another dose and your mood improves further. Each additional dose you take makes you feel more and more happy. In this scenario, knowing exactly where you cross the line from "lowered depression" (ie. – feeling happier) to "high" is very important. Apart from this, all you will have to go on is whether or not you are complying with the doctor's instructions regarding dose and timing of dose.

Before you go...

If you enjoyed this book, check out my author page on Amazon for more.

Also, if you think that others could benefit from the information I have provided, please consider leaving an honest review here on Amazon.

Appendix 1 - Pharmacogenetics and liver enzymes

As mentioned in the book, one of the most important factors in your response to different drugs is the status of each individual type of enzyme. These enzymes (and in particular, *CYP2D6*) largely dictate how much of your dose is absorbed and how quickly it is eliminated from the body.

Fortunately, in most countries it is relatively easy to have your enzyme function quantified, providing you and your doctor with an invaluable tool to guide the choice of medication. Some drugs are metabolised by other enzymes (such as *CYP3A4*) and some drugs are not even metabolised in the liver. In addition, some drugs are actually pro-drugs, which are inert/inactive until they undergo metabolism via one of these enzymes. Examples of these include codeine and tramadol.

Each of these enzymes belongs to a family. For example, CYP2D6 belongs to the CYP2 family and CPY3A4 belongs to the CYP3 family.

One other thing to bear in mind however, is the fact that, depending on the country, its healthcare system or your own individual insurance status, this test can be expensive. If you can't afford to have it done, it is not a crucial aspect of your pharmacotherapy, however it can certainly help your doctor create a more targeted treatment from the outset.

I initially planned on writing this part of the appendix from scratch, however in the process I discovered a fantastic overview on PubMed. So you can either click that link or read my edited version below, if you are reading the print version of this book. While this overview was written in the context of the breast cancer drug *Tamoxifen*, the principles hold for antidepressants.

Introduction to CYP2D6 and *CYP2D6* testing

Pharmacogenetic testing and the use of testing in clinical practice is a relatively new, evolving and complex topic. This short summary provides an introduction to the basic concepts that need to be considered in relation to cytochrome P450 2D6 (CYP2D6) and *CYP2D6* testing.

Enzymes, genes and pharmacogenetics

Differences in the response of individuals to the same drug at the same dose may occur as a result of interindividual differences in enzymes (e.g. CYP2D6) responsible for metabolising the drug. These differences may be inherited and occur as a result of differences in the genes (e.g. *CYP2D6*) that encode the enzyme.

In humans, each gene is composed of two alleles, one inherited from each parent, and a person may have two copies of the same allele (homozygous) or one copy of two different alleles (heterozygous). Alleles that differ from the normal or common form are known as polymorphisms [variant (*vt*)], while a normal allele is referred to as wild type (*wt*). It is from these differences that an individual's genotype is derived, for example the homozygous *wt* (i.e. *wt/wt*) genotype.

A phenotype is the observable physical trait of an organism, which, in pharmacogenetics, relates to an individual's reaction to a drug, usually as a result of the way in which the drug is metabolised. The phenotype is largely determined by the overall genetic make-up of a person, although it may also be influenced by environmental factors (e.g. diet and smoking).

The cytochrome P450 (CYP450) enzyme system, to which CYP2D6 belongs, has been identified as a major metabolic pathway for many drugs and a source of interindividual variability in patient response. It is believed to play a prominent role in the way in which tamoxifen (TAM) is metabolised and thus may explain differences in responses in individual patients to the same dose as it is known that TAM is metabolised to its active metabolites (which are thought to affect patient response, rather than TAM itself) by a number of CYP450 enzymes (including CYP2D6).

Based on studies that have examined the urinary metabolic ratios of drugs such as debrisoquine and/or dextromethorphan to their metabolites (4-hydroxydebrisoquine and dextrorphan, respectively), an association between *CYP2D6* genotypes (genetic make-up) and phenotypes (response to treatment) is believed to exist. It is thus also believed that patients experiencing a normal response at a normal dose of TAM would be *CYP2D6* extensive metabolisers (EMs). These individuals are thought to be homozygous for the *wt* allele. Patients experiencing reduced clinical effects owing to deficient alleles are referred to as poor metabolisers (PMs) and are thought to be homozygous (and possibly heterozygous) for the *vt* allele.

However, there are a number of different *vt* alleles, some which result in decreased enzyme activity and others that result in a complete lack of enzyme activity (i.e. the differing extent to which the drug is metabolised). PMs must possess at least one of these complete lack of function alleles (e.g. *4;).

Genotyping for *CYP2D6*

There is growing anticipation that genotyping for CYP2D6 may be used to assist in treatment decision-making. A number of these tests have been developed and are described in the literature, and have been used for a wide range of drugs and diseases, not just TAM and breast cancer. However, not all tests will be the same.

Appendix 2 - Tricyclic (TCA) drugs and their mechanism of action via binding affinities

I am not normally one for lazy Wikipedia cut & paste jobs, however despite my intention of creating my own table, I realised that the one on Wikipedia was already perfect. So I begrudgingly include it below. You can also see a live version on the Wikipedia TCA page.

Compound ◆	SERT ◆	NET ◆	DAT ◆	5-HT$_{1A}$ ◆	5-HT$_{2A}$ ◆	5-HT$_{2C}$ ◆	5-HT$_6$ ◆	5-HT$_7$ ◆	α$_1$ ◆	α$_2$ ◆	D$_2$ ◆	H$_1$ ◆	mACh ◆
Amitriptyline	3.13	22.4	4,430	320	24	6.15	103.1	114	26	815	1,230	1.03	13.8
Butriptyline	1,360	5,100	3,940	7,000	380	?	?	?	570	4,800	?	1.1	35
Clomipramine	0.21	45.85	2,605	>10,000	35.5	64.6	53.8	127	3.2	525	119.8	31	37
Desipramine	179	2.27	3,190	>10000	315	?	?	?	115	6,350	1,561	45.4	232.6
Dosulepin	8.6	46	5,310	4,004	258	?	?	?	470	2,400	?	4	63.6
Doxepin	68	29.5	12,100	276	27	8.8	136	?	24	1,185	1,380	0.21	81.4
Imipramine	1.6	51.67	8,500	>10,000	118.67	120	190.3	1000	61	3,150	1,310	24	68
Iprindole	1,620	1,262	6,530	2,800	217	206	?	?	2,300	8,600	?	130	2,100
Lofepramine	70	5.4	18,000	4,600	200	?	?	?	100	2,700	2,000	360	67
Nortriptyline	16.5	1.65	5,000	302	43	8.5	148	?	58	2,265	1,885	8.2	94
Protriptyline	19.6	1.41	2,100	3,800	70	?	?	?	130	6,600	2,300	60	25
Trimipramine	149	2,450	3,780	8,000	32	?	?	?	24	680	180	0.27	58

To understand the above, there are things I will need to explain, as these types of binding affinity charts can be confusing at first glance.

Firstly, the acronyms –

SERT – The serotonin transporter. Reuptake inhibitors block SERT

NET – Noradrenaline/norepinephrine transporter. SNRIs and TCAs block it.

DAT – Dopamine transporter. Ditto.

5-HT – Serotonin receptors. The smaller numbers (1A, 2A etc) represent the different sub-types

α$_1$ & α$_2$ - Alpha-adrenal receptors

D$_2$ - D2 dopamine receptor

H1 - H1 histamine receptor

mAChR - Muscarinic acetylcholine receptor

Next, let's look at what the numbers mean. Each of these values is known as a binding affinity which, for the purpose of this explanation, should be considered as a measure of potency.

However where people sometimes trip up is how they interpret the numbers, because naturally you would expect that the higher the number, the more potency. However, surprisingly, the inverse is true, so the lower the number, the more potently that drug binds to the target receptor. Binding affinity is expressed as Ki in nM, which is essentially a representation of how many receptors the drug binds to under a particular experimental condition.

Note that this is a gross simplification of what is a hugely complicated process, however as I assume you are reading this to learn just enough to be able to understand different drugs and their effects, and not for the purposes of obtaining a degree in pharmacology, I think this is the clearest way to explain this topic.

Also you should bear in mind that this is simpler when we are talking about agonists which bind and activate a receptor. However if we are referring to an antagonist, it would be more accurate to say that the higher the binding affinity, the more the drug can prevent the receptor from becoming activated.

Looking at the binding affinities of various drugs can help you gain an understanding of which ones might suit your own neurochemistry. For example, fluoxetine has a Ki of 1.0 nM, whereas paroxetine is 0.08 nM. So clearly paroxetine is a significantly more potent drug for inhibiting the reuptake of serotonin. However you also must bear in mind the dosage. For example, fluoxetine is obviously weaker than paroxetine, however if you increase the dosage of fluoxetine and keep the paroxetine dosage steady, at a certain point the drugs should theoretically become equipotent.

However the complexity doesn't end there, as there will be person to person differences in how they metabolise drugs. So in theory, you could have someone who experiences the same net SERT inhibition for both fluoxetine and paroxetine, as they are able to absorb more of fluoxetine or perhaps their liver clears paroxetine faster.

So say you have compared SSRI versus SSRI, you may then wish to look at SSRI versus TCA. If you look at the above chart, it doesn't take long to see that clomipramine is by far the most serotonergic of all TCAs at 0.21 nM Ki. However let's assume that you think you would benefit from something a little milder in terms of serotonergic effects and with some NRI added. In this case, amitriptyline could be an option. This is one of the reasons why amitriptyline is the most commonly used TCA, with a good balance between serotonin and noradrenaline, along with some sleep-promoting H1 blocking (antihistamine) action.

Appendix 3 – Reboxetine – Big Pharma's Shame

You, like just about everyone I talk to who is not from a medical background, may not be aware of the fact that drug companies are under no obligation to release all the data they have collected in the clinical trials they sponsor. They can choose which data to release and which data not to release. I will give you one guess which data they bury.

When the team from IQWiG contacted Pfizer to ask for all the data, they initially stonewalled, saying they would only provide "those data that from our point of view are suited for a benefit assessment of Edronax". Yes, you read that correctly. Pfizer thought that they should only have to provide the data which they had decided would be "suited for a benefit assessment".

Things became a little murky at that point (I have tried to piece the story together via the BMJ's own publications and newspaper articles released in the wake of the trial). However those plucky souls at IQWiG apparently worked out that Pfizer had buried 74% of the data! Then, after some back and forth (perhaps lawyer to lawyer – this part of the process is unclear), IQWiG staff were somehow able to coax the remaining data out of Pfizer, enabling them to complete the review with the full picture, rather than the picture Pfizer decided we should see.

So I bet you are on the edge of your seat, right?[40]

I imagine you wouldn't be particularly surprised to learn that clinical trial papers are very, very dry. They use such ambiguous phraseology that sometimes it takes a while to work out whether the study was positive or negative. This is largely to convey a sense of objectivity, so that "opinion" doesn't overshadow the data. Against this general backdrop, the BMJ's findings were about as close to a *smackdown* as you will find in this field. When referring to certain findings, the IQWiG team's tone was dripping with scorn, verging on outrage.

To cut to the chase, the study found that -

"Our analysis of a comprehensive evidence base of published and unpublished trials of reboxetine compared with placebo or SSRIs in adults with major depressive disorder indicates that reboxetine is, overall, an ineffective and potentially harmful antidepressant. Published evidence on reboxetine has been substantially affected by publication bias, underlining the urgent need for mandatory publication of clinical trial data, including data on older agents."

Regarding Pfizer's obfuscation, the reviewers again pulled no punches –

*"A substantial proportion of patient data (74%) had not been previously published…For both benefit outcomes, **the addition of unpublished data changed the superiority of reboxetine versus placebo shown in published data to a non-significant difference**"*

---

[40] Who says you can't have a rollicking yarn in a book about antidepressants!

and also changed the non-significant difference between reboxetine and SSRIs to an inferiority of reboxetine...Comparison of the published data with the full dataset (published and unpublished) showed that the published data overestimated the beneficial effect of reboxetine compared with placebo by 99-115% and of reboxetine compared with SSRIs by 19-23%."

The IQWiG and the BMJ should be commended for taking a stand against one of Big Pharma's dirty little secrets. It is not every day you see a respected journal accuse one of the world's largest pharmaceutical companies of cherry picking the data to give a false impression that reboxetine is effective as an antidepressant. The reviewers also used reboxetine's rather extreme example to illustrate a broader issue -

"Our difficulties in retrieving unpublished trial data and our results of the comparison between published and previously unpublished trials are a further example of publication bias, a problem that has been known in clinical research for decades...Such bias, including industry sponsorship bias, has frequently been identified in research on antidepressants...For example, Turner et al published a comparison of FDA reviews of placebo controlled antidepressant trials and matching publications, which showed that, overall, published trials overestimated effect sizes by 32%"

When the BMJ study came out, it literally sent shockwaves through the medical research and government health policy communities. It's not often a meta-analysis is reported in Time, Newsweek, Forbes, The Guardian, Scientific American and The Daily Mail UK. One of the reasons for this is the fact that (at least initially) reboxetine had performed well in animal models and had pharmacodynamics which should, in theory, help treat depression. This issue was captured well by an article in Scientific American –

"And this is a rough moment for scientists studying depression. Why? Because reboxetine works beautifully in our animal models. It's practically a poster-child antidepressant. It produces acute effects in tests such as forced-swim tests and tail-suspension tests (which use changes in struggle as a measure of antidepressant efficacy). It produces neurogenesis in the hippocampus, which is thought to be correlated with antidepressant effects...But it doesn't work in patients. And patients are what matters. Now, scientists are stuck with a difficult question: What went wrong? This is more than just an issue with an antidepressant that didn't work, it's an issue with the tests we are using to study depression. How effective are they, really? Are we in fact modeling the right things? Do the tail-suspension test and forced-swim test detect antidepressant activity after all? And if they aren't detecting antidepressant activity, what are they actually doing? What does this mean for both the neurochemical theory of depression and the neurogenesis theory? Reboxetine affects both but still has no clinical effect. Does this mean that both of these theories are wrong? Or does it mean that they are incomplete? And where, exactly, do we go from here?"

The take-away message here is that we need to build an understanding of a drug's efficacy by looking in a holistic way, including –

- Binding affinities to demonstrate (even in basic terms) the drug's pharmacology
- The results of various rodent trials
- Real world user feedback
- The clinical experience of doctors
- The drug's statistically-defined efficacy in human trials, based on all the data – not just the data the drug company wants you to see

Regarding this last point, you will be happy to learn that an organisation called AllTrials is trying to get this situation rectified by convincing governments to compel drug companies to release all clinical trial data on "all trials", irrespective of whether the drug was released or not. AllTrials is an initiative of Bad Science, which is run by well-known author Dr Ben Goldacre, with support from the BMJ, Centre for Evidence-based Medicine, Cochrane Collaboration and many other organisations. In the US, Darmouth's School of Medicine is championing the cause (Here is the complete list of supporters).

You can do your part as well by signing the petition on the site calling for drug companies to publish all trials.

Appendix 4 – The Ian Hickie agomelatine controversy

The following was published in <u>The Australian Doctor</u>, in 2012 –

One of Australia's most high-profile psychiatrists has come under fire for "overstating" the benefits of a new antidepressant that critics say is ineffective and potentially unsafe. A series of letters to the *Lancet* Friday accused Professor Ian Hickie of promoting the strength of evidence on agomelatine [Valdoxan], while downplaying safety concerns. They also took aim at the drug company ties of Professor Hickie and colleague Associate Professor Naomi Rogers, suggesting these had contributed to their "subjective" and "inappropriate" appraisal of the drug.

Professors Hickie and Rogers, who rejected the claims, had recently authored a Lancet review on the new class of melatonin-based antidepressants, focusing on agomelatine. They said the drug had "clinically significant" effects, with similar short-term efficacy to venlafaxine, fluoxetine, and sertraline. They concluded its favourable safety profile and positive effects on circadian function meant it "might occupy a unique place" in the management of some patients.

However, their article was dissected by six scathing letters to the journal. Several suggested the data had been cherry-picked and not systematically appraised. In one letter, French doctors said that half the placebo-controlled trials of agomelatine had been negative, and others "too weak" to draw conclusions on efficacy. In another, a US psychiatrist said the rare risk of liver toxicity with agomelatine – "a unique safety issue among antidepressant drugs"- was not highlighted in published studies.

Professor Jon Jureidini and Melissa Raven, Adelaide-based members of Healthy Skepticism, said in a third letter the article's summary contained "unjustified and misleading conclusions", and raised concerns over possible conflicts of interest. "The Lancet's publication of this flawed paper will undoubtedly validate marketing of Valdoxan, and we are curious to see how many paid Valdoxan advertisements will be published in Elsevier journals," they wrote. However, Professors Hickie and Rogers stood by their review, saying it had been "balanced and independent". Many of the issues, such as the challenge of demonstrating clear efficacy over placebo, were common to all antidepressants, they said, and changes in liver function tests were well recognised with agomelatine, and reflected in monitoring recommendations. They said their paper had been commissioned by the Lancet, was neither initiated nor supported financially by Valdoxan manufacturer Servier, and expressed only the authors' opinions. Agomelatine is available on private script in Australia, having twice been rejected for PBS listing.